Don't Diet!
Just Think
And
Get Thin

Don't Diet!
Just Think
And
Get Thin

You must first win the battle of the mind before you can win the battle of the bulge.

George A. Diamond

A & C Publishing
AC-Publishing.com

Published 2011 by A & C Publishing
© Copyright 2011 George A. Diamond
AC-Publishing.com
2nd Edition

ISBN-13: 978-0-615-41515-4

Dedication

I dedicate this book to my brother-in-law George who died at the young age of 48.

Acknowledgments

Writing a book involves a lot of time and work. Therefore, I would like to thank some people who helped make this book a reality.

First of all, I want to thank my wife and children for their support while writing this book.

I want to thank my parents for their guidance and encouragement while I was growing up.

I would like to thank Bill Kleist for designing the cover.

Lastly, I want to thank a friend of mine, Andrew Owens, for his encouragement while I was in the weight-loss process and while writing this book.

Contents

Introduction

"The greatest pleasure in life is doing what people say you cannot do."

Walter Bagehot

"Imprisoned in every fat man, a thin one is wildly signaling to be let out."

Cyril Connolly

First I want to make one thing clear. I have no medical degrees, no health certificates hanging on my wall, and I am not a personal trainer. The one thing I do have is results in losing weight, getting physically fit, and keeping it off. The 50 pounds I lost in 4 months and the five years and counting of maintenance of that new weight are my credentials. This book will take you down the same path I took so that you too can accomplish your weight-loss goal, if you choose to do so. This book will allow you to follow in my footsteps to get down to your desired weight and stay there. This book is not about dieting but about changing your thinking and your attitudes towards eating, health, and fitness. Once this is accomplished, losing weight and maintaining a healthy lifestyle will follow.

I have found that most people move from diet to diet looking for the magic pill, the new thing, the quick thing, that will allow them to lose weight without doing anything different. That is not what this book is about. This is not a diet book or a quick-and-easy way-to-lose-weight book. It is a systematic approach to losing weight by changing the way you think about some things. Remember, it is your thinking that keeps you from overeating or snacking. It is your thinking that motivates you to exercise. Change your thinking and the rest falls into place.

The average life span of a person is 73-77 years. This is too short of a time not to live healthy. It starts with something you can control: your weight and your fitness. It all comes down to the choices you make daily. No matter what you think, you are in control. This book will outline how to unleash the power of your mind to take and keep control of your weight. The only question is, "Are you willing to make it happen?" Good. Then let's get started.

Step 1
Embrace Your True Reality
(Your Ah-Ha Moment)

"Until I am ready to lose weight, I cannot see how fat I am."

Mason Cooley

About 15 years ago I gained a couple of pounds and did not even realize it. The next year I gained a few more pounds. The year after that, I gained a few more pounds and realized one thing. I realized that my wife had shrunk my clothes. That was the only answer. So I went out and bought some new clothes. The following year I gained a few more pounds and this went on for years. It went on for years because I was in denial. I was unwilling to admit I had gained weight. See, it took me years to become overweight. I did not become large overnight. It was a slow process. My weight gain snuck up on me.

There were times when someone would mention that I looked like I had gained weight. When this happened, I would sometimes make an excuse by saying I was getting older. Alternatively, I would make a joke and say that it was all muscle, or I would joke it off by saying that my wife was a great cook (this is true, by the way). However, deep down, I really didn't think I was overweight. Yes, I knew I had gained a couple of pounds, but I never saw myself as overweight. I did not ever think I had a weight problem. I had a false sense of reality, and I was looking at my weight through rose-colored glasses.

"The definition of insanity is doing the same thing and expecting different results."

Albert Einstein

This Albert Einstein quote is one of my favorites because it speaks to human nature. Too often people (including me and probably you) feel that they can get different results without changing a thing. I wanted to lose a couple of pounds, but I did not want to change what I was doing

3

to make it happen, because as I mentioned earlier, I did not think I had a problem. If you want to change your weight, you need to change what you are doing. This is the bottom line. I will use this quote throughout this book because I feel it is a powerful reminder of what you need to do (change your thinking, change your beliefs, change your attitudes, and change your habits concerning health, weight, and fitness) to change your results.

As I mentioned earlier, I had a false sense of reality. I was looking at my weight through rose-colored glasses. The first thing I did was to take the rose-colored glasses off and see myself as overweight and admit it. When that happened, I embraced my true reality. The first step in losing weight is to embrace your true reality.

You might still wonder why you need to embrace your true reality. The answer is simple. It is impossible to lose weight if you refuse to admit that you have a problem. That is why it is important to identify and admit that you have a weight problem and are living an unhealthy lifestyle. It is about removing the filters that you see yourself through (your rose-colored glasses). They are the mental filters that keep you overweight, that cloud your perspective and give you a false reality.

Like drugs and alcohol, being overweight is a problem and food is your addiction (not in all cases). This problem is sustained through bad eating habits. In most drug and alcohol programs, the first step is to admit you have a problem. This is the first step in solving it. In losing weight it's no different. Most people will admit they could lose a couple of pounds but deny that it is a real problem that they must solve. True reality is being totally honest with yourself. The greatest threat to yourself is to ignore or deny your true reality. If you have a true understanding of your weight situation, you know where you are and where you want to be. You must see your reality as it currently is here and now. It is only by seeing the reality of your weight problem that you can begin to move forward towards being thinner and fitter. Remember not to sacrifice your future for a false reality. Looking at the true current reality of your weight problem is one of the hardest things to do, but it is a necessary step in the process. You can only make changes in your lifestyle when you know where you currently are.

Picture it like going to a mall and looking at the directory. It makes no sense to see where you want to go if you don't find the **YOU ARE HERE** tag. That is why the first thing that needs to happen is for us to see ourselves in our true reality. That is what I like to call the *Ah-Ha Moment.*

My reality came one day as I was standing in front of the mirror with my shirt off, brushing my teeth before I went to bed. (Please don't visualize this. It was not a pretty sight.) Usually I would have my shirt on when I brushed my teeth, but for some reason this time I did not. My belly was jiggling all over the place and I just about got sick. I stood there and really looked at myself and thought, "How did I let myself get this way?" This was my *Ah-Ha Moment.* Until then I ignored my weight. I also justified my weight by saying, "Well, I don't look so bad even with a few extra pounds." I defended, excused, and ignored my poor decisions. Most people live in their own false reality (me included). They justify, blame, and excuse their bad choices. Your body will do what your head and brain tell it to. Your car doesn't just turn into the drive-thru of a fast-food restaurant. Your brain tells it. That doesn't make you a bad person. You just make the wrong choices, whether you are aware of it or not.

It reminds me of an ostrich that puts its head in a hole when a lion comes to eat it. It thinks that if it doesn't see the lion, then obviously the lion doesn't see it. For me, it wasn't until that moment in the bathroom that my true reality was shown to me, and I could accept it. I then realized that if I was going to change my weight, I was going to have to be willing to make some changes in my life. What is your true reality? Are you willing to see it and accept it? How do you know if you are in self-denial?

Below are six ways to check if you may be in self-denial:
1. You say to yourself, "I'm not overweight. I just gained a few pounds."
2. You say, "I can lose weight any time I want to."
3. You say, "I would lose weight but I don't like to exercise."
4. You say, "I am going to lose weight after (a particular date)."
5. You tell yourself, "My thinking is exactly where it needs to be to lose weight, even though I have not lost a pound."
6. You say, "I eat all the right things and can't lose weight. It must

be my metabolism." (This may be true but have a doctor confirm it.)

If you are overweight and not actively losing weight weekly, you may be denying that you have a weight problem. There is also a good chance that if you do realize and accept your weight problem, you still may be denying that your future will be affected negatively by it.

I think that stories are a good way to teach, so I will tell a few of them throughout this book. The first story I want to tell you displays a form of denial I have run into on more than one occasion.

As an entrepreneur, I own multiple businesses. One of the businesses I own is an IT company that supplies computer services to small and medium-sized businesses. A few months ago a client of mine told me that I had inspired him. He said that if I could lose weight, he could do it too. He asked me what I did to lose it. I told him, "*You need to win the battle of the mind before you can win the battle of the bulge.*" His response in a very confident tone was, "I already won that battle." I didn't say anything, but I thought that if he had already won that battle, he would already be thin. Well, a half hour later at lunch he proved himself wrong. He was eating a giant order of fried chicken, french fries, rolls, and coleslaw brought in from the nearby fast-food restaurant. I could not let this one pass by without some teaching. I walked by him, patted his shoulder and in a joking manner said, "Well, I guess you lost the battle of the mind." Then I kept walking, not waiting for a response.

I did not say this to embarrass him or to be mean-spirited. I said it to make him THINK. Had I stayed to talk after making the comment, he would have become defensive and would have had to come up with a rebuttal. By leaving, I forced him to think about what I said. It worked, because later in the day he came to me to discuss it further. He also admitted during our conversation that he was not as ready mentally for the battle as he thought.

In this case, his reality told him that he needed to lose weight, but it also told him that he was already mentally prepared to take on the task. His warped reality was not in line with his true reality. Winning the battle of the mind also includes winning the tough battle of self-denial,

6

and what you don't want to do is to let denial set your future. This story illustrates that denial can occur in a variety of ways. The key is to recognize it.

"The greatest fool is one who fools himself."

Unknown Author

Earlier we looked at six ways you can tell that you are battling self-denial. Below are five questions that will give you the reasons behind that denial, if you answer them honestly. Having an understanding through knowing **why** is an important part of the weight-loss process.

Ask yourself the following questions:
1) Why am I not thin and in shape?
2) Why haven't I been able to lose weight and get in shape?
3) Why can't I lose weight and get in shape?
4) Why don't I lose weight and get in shape?
5) Why can't I start now?

If you answer these questions with anything other than, "I just don't want to lose weight," you are probably making excuses, placing blame somewhere else, justifying the poor decisions you made in the past, and deceiving yourself.

This may sound harsh but I am here to help you get your head in the right place, not tiptoe around the problem, and definitely not to tell you that it is not your fault.

I want you to look in the mirror with your shirt off, and if you don't like what you see, change it. If your mid-section jiggles when you brush your teeth, do something about it. If you look in the mirror and don't like what you see, but you start justifying why you can't lose weight, you are just fooling yourself.

"A wish changes nothing. A decision changes everything."

Unknown Author

Once you realize that you need to lose weight, the next step is to decide to do something about it and find an intense reason or reasons for losing weight. In other words, you need to find your motivation. You need to find your **Reason Why**.

"Not to decide is to decide."

Harvey Cox

A lot of people I talk to say that they need to lose weight, but they don't truly see and understand what it means to be overweight. That is their false reality. Also, I have learned over the years that people tend to do not what they need to do but only what they truly want to do. What they want to do is to avoid discomfort which they associate with losing weight and getting fit. That is why they avoid it like the plague.

So decide once and for all to do this and let's find your motivation. Remember, if you are overweight or obese, you are a ticking time bomb. It is just a matter of time until you explode. Only you can decide to make the proper changes in your life for a healthy lifestyle. The right decision is usually not always the easy one, but in this case it has great rewards. In this case it is all about the quality and length of your life. Let's find your **Reason Why**.

Step 2
Give Yourself a "Reason Why"
(Your Motivation)

*"So oftentimes it happens that we live our lives in chains,
and we never even know we have the key."*

The Eagles

In the previous section I talked about finding your true reality, and you
do that by battling self-denial. When this happens you will have your
Ah-Ha Moment. Like I said in the previous section, it happened to me
one night when I walked into the bathroom with my shirt off to brush
my teeth and my belly was jiggling all over the place. Usually I would
go into the bathroom with my shirt on, so I really never noticed it
before. However, this time was different. I looked at myself in the
mirror and said, "What happened? How did I let myself get like this?
How did I get this way?" Bingo, I just had my **Ah-Ha Moment**.

Once you have had your **Ah-Ha Moment,** the next step is to find your
motivation**,** or as I like to say, you need to find your **Reason Why**.

Motivation is the internal fuel and fire that drives you to towards a
goal. It is the burning desire that drives you to go after a goal with
passion, with intensity, with commitment and with determination.
Motivation is the fuel that will continue to drive you through the ups
and downs of the weight-loss process. Motivation is internal (self-
motivation). It is not external (someone else motivating you). That is
the reason why all outside motivations are temporary and do not work.
External motivation can get you going for the short term, but it will not
keep you that way. This is because once the external motivator leaves,
the motivation will disappear. In other words, no one can motivate you
but yourself, not even me. Neither I nor anyone else can motivate you,
and I am here not to motivate you, but to educate you, so that you can
learn to motivate yourself.

Only you can motivate you, and having a significant **Reason Why** is
mandatory to losing weight. If you have tried to lose weight in the

9

past, and you haven't, it is because you do not have a strong enough desire. You do not have a big enough *Reason Why*. Your *Reason Why* has to be strong enough to drive you emotionally. It has to be able to light a fire underneath you. It has to be something that you can keep in your head all the time, through the good times and the bad times, through the successes and the failures of moving through the weight-loss process. Your *Reason Why* has to be strong, and you need to fuel that fire from within daily.

The great thing is that you can learn to motivate yourself. This can be done by learning what gets you going, and it is different for everyone. Remember, you will only lose weight when you really truly want to and are ready, not when you need to. I talk to a lot of people who tell me they want to lose weight but never do anything about it. This is because although they may realize that they need to lose weight, they don't actually want to lose weight. Needing, wanting, and doing are three different things.

One of the things you can do to motivate yourself into getting thinner and fitter is to have a dream, or the opposite of a dream, which is called a dread. This is your *Reason Why*. This may sound strange, but finding your *Reason Why* is, in reality, focusing on something other than the process itself. It can be used to fuel your motivation. It is the driving force that will keep you exercising and eating right, even when you don't feel like it. It will also be the driving force in helping you to monitor your eating. So, the question is, "Do you have a dream or a dread?" What is your *Reason Why*? What is the reason you want to lose weight? What is the reason that will drive you through the ups and downs? What is the reason that will keep you focused and keep your head in the game? People will lose weight for one of two reasons: Either they lose weight for something they will get out of it (a dream) or because of something they don't want or are trying to stay away from (a dread) like the health problems that being overweight or obese brings. Which category do you fall under? What is it that will move you emotionally? Whatever your driving force is, find or create it and then focus on it, all the time.

Did you ever get up and go to work in the morning, even though you didn't feel like it? Why is that? It's because of what you get out of it, namely a certain standard of living, a home to live in, food on the table, a car, etc. It's what motivates you to get up in the morning and go to work. You can look at losing weight the same way. You can look at what you will get out of it and use that to motivate you. You can look at things like enhanced mobility, looking younger, feeling better, the envy of others who are heavy, a longer and healthier life, decreased wear and tear on your body, the ability to enjoy your family more because you are healthy, more energy, clearer thinking, a more positive attitude, etc.

If you have not been able to lose weight in the past, there is a reason: It is because your dream, dread, or *Reason Why* is not big enough to fuel the motivation within you. When your dream, dread, or *Reason Why* is large enough, you will find a way to lose the weight you want. Find a reason that will emotionally fire you up and keep you that way. Alter your thinking so that the misery of staying the same weight is worse than the misery of change, and you will have the key to losing weight. It will be as good as done. When you find your *Reason Why*, you will find the time and create the energy and passion, and you will do it.

If you don't have a **Reason Why**, now is the time to find one and start moving to achieve it. Today is the day to make the time, start believing you can do it, and put the action behind it. Like the Nike commercial says, "*Just do it.*" Start each day with a plan that will give you the intense focus needed to protect you against destructive eating.

However, if you have no motivation, no dream, no dread, and no reason why, there will always be something that will stop you from succeeding in losing the weight you desire. Having the time will constantly be a problem, and things will come up that will give you an excuse to make the wrong choices, like skipping exercise and eating poorly. This will cause the opposite effect and the pounds will continue to accumulate. Years will continue to pass and your health will diminish and the pains of regret will settle in. The pains of regret include wishing you had not overeaten, thereby sacrificing the future for the now. Regret will also include wishing you had done something to lose weight.

Let's explore some ways you can dig deep inside to motivate yourself. As I mentioned before, the first thing you need to do is find your *Reason Why*.

My *Reason Why* was created right after I had my *Ah-Ha Moment*. I just had the teeth-brushing experience and went to check on my two boys before I went to bed. I checked in on my younger boy and then checked in on my older boy. My motivation hit me like a brick upside my head. I went back in and looked at my boys and thought to myself, "I want to watch them grow up. I want to be healthy enough to play ball with them, bike with them, and jog with them. I want to dance at their weddings. I want to be around to watch them get married." I realized that I was on a road, going in a direction that did not have a good ending. Just then a rush of strong emotions came flooding at me, and I knew I needed to change the road I was traveling on and get on the road to lower weight and fitness.

I walked back in the bathroom, looked at myself square in the eyes and said to myself, "I am going to lose weight. It is done." I did not go into the bathroom and say, "I am going to try to lose weight and see what happens." I said, "I am going to lose weight. It is done." There was no question about it and no hesitation. How I was going to do it, I didn't know, but it is done, and that has been fueling my fire since. I still think about it daily, and it continues to drive me because I found my *Reason Why*.

My question to you is this: What is your *Reason Why*? What is your motivation? What will get and keep you emotionally fired up? Once you find your reason, place it on the refrigerator, write it down on the bathroom mirror with a dry-erase marker, and use it as your daily reminder(s) of the battle you are fighting, the battle you will win, the battle against the bulge.

A few tools that can help you find your *Reason Why* are the worksheets below. They will help you organize your thoughts in a logical manner and show you the road you need to take.

Let's start by answering the following questions. The answers need to get you emotionally charged. If they don't, you haven't found your *Reason Why*.

What are the risks associated with <u>not</u> losing weight?

Rank them as you perceive them from Most Important to Least Important.

Most Important   1)

                              2)

                              3)

                              4)

                              5)

                              6)

                              7)

                              8)

                              9)

Least Important   10)

What are the risks in losing weight?

Biggest Risk   1)

                           2)

                           3)

                           4)

                           5)

                           6)

                           7)

                           8)

                           9)

Smallest Risk   10)

What are the advantages of losing weight?

Biggest Advantage   1)

2)

3)

4)

5)

6)

7)

8)

9)

Least Important   10)
Advantage

What are the advantages of <u>not</u> losing weight?

Biggest Advantage   1)

2)

3)

4)

5)

6)

7)

8)

9)

Least Important   10)
Advantage

What are the disadvantages of <u>not</u> losing weight?

Biggest Disadvantage 1)

2)

3)

4)

5)

6)

7)

8)

9)

Least Urgent   10)
Disadvantage

Make a list of the things that are important to you in your life. Is it your family, success, relationships, power, choices, freedom, control, or money? Make a list of the top ten in priority order.

What is important to you in your life?

Most Important   1)

2)

3)

4)

5)

6)

7)

8)

9)

Tenth-Most   10)
Important

Review the last list you just made. Can you have any of these things and enjoy them without your health? If you lost some weight and got fitter, would that support your priorities? Can you have success and enjoy it without your health? Let's look at that a minute. If you are not healthy, your concentration and focus are greatly diminished. Your energy level is generally lower. Your attitude is usually not as good as it could be. How can you possibly be successful with all this against you? I am not saying that if you are overweight you cannot be successful. What I am saying is that if you are overweight, you add extra challenges on the road to success. Therefore, if you value success, you need to value one of the underlying foundations of success: good health, which may be obtained and kept if you are thinner. Can you truly enjoy your family to the fullest without your health? Without your health, the list is meaningless.

I know a wealthy man who has cancer. He said he would start all over without a dime to get his health back. Nothing is as important as your health. The best way to change your thinking is to not only acknowledge this fact but also allow this to grab you emotionally so that you want to lose weight and become healthier.

However, if health is not at the top of your list, this may be why you are overweight. It is not important to you. The reality is that it must be at the top of your list if you want to enjoy the rest of the items on your list.

Another attitude that you need to develop is to become very dissatisfied about your current weight. Don't get depressed about it, but get excited and motivated that you have the ability to change it, if you desire.

I hope the answers to the questions above have helped clarify the priorities in your life. The key to losing weight is to focus on your **Reason Why** and not on the little inconveniences of the process.

Now that you have prioritized what is most important in your life, you need to connect that to being healthy, thin, and fit. To help you do this, let's fill out the worksheets below. The answers here should get you emotionally charged and help drive you in the right direction.

List how becoming thinner will help you with the things most important to you:

Biggest Way   1)

2)

3)

4)

5)

6)

7)

8)

9)

Smallest   10)

List how <u>not</u> losing weight affects those things most important to you:

Biggest Way   1)

                            2)

                            3)

                            4)

                            5)

                            6)

                            7)

                            8)

                            9)

Smallest   10)

The above worksheets form your reasons for losing weight.

If you still haven't found your **_Reason Why_**, here are a few things to think about. Remember that motivation is different for everyone:

- If you have young children or grandchildren, do you want to be around to see them grow into happy, healthy adults?
- Do it for your kids. People do more for their kids than themselves. Do it for them.
- If you have kids, look into their eyes and tell yourself that you want to be around to see them grow up.
- Kids tend to follow their parents. If they see you overeat, eat the wrong foods, and not exercise, they will follow. Are you setting a good example for your kids? Are you leading your family by example? I sometimes wonder if weight problems in families are just poor eating habits passed down from one generation to another and not genetics.
- If you are the breadwinner in the family, what would happen to your family if something happens to you? Are you being selfish by not keeping yourself as healthy, lean, and fit as you can? If you truly love your family wouldn't you want to live longer and healthier for them?
- Visit a nursing home and ask yourself how soon until you check in. Your health will determine it.
- At the time of writing this book, I saw a study from the University of Edinburgh in Scotland that said, "If you don't want to lose your mental function with aging, you need to be on a vigorous exercise program." In other words, if you want to lower the odds of dementia, you should exercise. Your mind is a terrible thing to lose.
- Reports indicate that weight loss may lower or prevent obesity-related diseases and catastrophes like:
  - Heart disease
  - Stroke
  - Hypertension
  - Type 2 diabetes
  - Cancer
  - High cholesterol or high triglycerides

- o Gallbladder disease
- o Sleep apnea and respiratory problems
- o Some cancers (e.g. endometrial, breast, colorectal, and kidney)
- o Osteoarthritis (degeneration of cartilage and bone of joints)
- o Complications during pregnancy
- o Menstrual irregularities
- o Excess body and facial hair
- o Stress incontinence
- o Psychological disorders, such as depression
- o Increased risk of surgical complications

- The ramifications of abusing your body may not be felt for years. If you are overweight and are still in good health, now is the time for action. Don't wait until there is a problem before you do something about it. By then it may be too late.
- Your body needs to last the rest of your life. It can be a healthy life or a sickly and very painful one. I am not saying that just because you are at a good weight you are guaranteed excellent health. What I am saying is that you optimize your chances of having fewer health problems if you are at a healthy weight. When it comes to the quality of your life, play the odds, lose weight, and play to win.
- Over and over the experts say that being overweight or obese increases your risk of the diseases listed above. They also say that if you are overweight or obese, you can delay or prevent some of these diseases by losing 5 to 10 percent of your weight. What is that telling you?
- Is trading the quality of your life worth having the fast-food lunches, chips, beer, or seconds at dinner?
- What is your future worth?
- What is your family's future worth?
- If you are single, tell yourself that you want to make yourself more attractive to a future partner. Don't get bitter, get thinner.
- If you are older, tell yourself that you want to live a long, healthy and independent life.
- Do you have a dream? Do you have a dream of wearing that swimsuit, getting into that dress, having rock-hard abs?

- I have never ever heard any statistics that say that being overweight, obese or out of shape helps you live longer and healthier. Get the point.
- Would you like to enjoy your family more? Do you think that if you are feeling better you can enjoy your family more? Sure you can. You can enjoy things more if you are feeling better. Do you think you would feel better if you lost weight and got fit? Of course you would. So lose weight, get fit, and enjoy your family more.
- Do you want more energy? If you lose weight you will have greater energy, you will feel better, and you will be able to accomplish a lot more.
- Do you want to get around better? It is a lot easier to get in and out of chairs, get in and out of your car, and walk up and down the stairs if you become thinner.
- Do you want a feeling of accomplishment? You will experience a great feeling of accomplishment when you lose weight and get fit.
- Do you want to feel comfortable in chairs? When I was heavier I felt constricted in theater chairs and in airplane seats. Public seats are not made for overweight people. If you are tired of feeling restricted and uncomfortable, do something about it!
- Would you like to save money? How would you like to save money on clothes, food, medical bills, and prescriptions?
- Would you like not having to spend your time waiting in doctors' offices and hospital rooms?
- Do you want to look great in that dress? Do you want to look good in that pair of shorts? Do you want to be able to wear shorts at all?
- Do you want to be active in your 80s and 90s?
- Do you want to end up in a wheelchair or using a walker before your time?
- Do you want to travel to Europe when you retire or travel back and forth to the hospital? The choice is yours. It starts with your weight.
- Do you want to look younger? You'll be amazed at the years you can cut off your looks by just losing weight.
- Do you want to feel younger? Do you want to be healthier?

- Do you want to have a better attitude? When you look good and feel great, you naturally have a better attitude.
- Do you want to avoid, eliminate, or reduce high blood pressure, diabetes, or high cholesterol?
- Do you want to reduce the chances of a heart attack or a stroke?
- If you have to go in for surgery, would you like to reduce complications? The better in shape you're in, the easier the surgery should go and the quicker your body can respond and heal itself.
- Do you want to stop fearing the scale?
- Do you want to stop fearing the doctor because he or she is going to tell you to lose weight?
- Do you want to be able to look at yourself in a full-length mirror and smile?
- Do you want to like looking at photos of yourself?
- Would you like to do some of the things that you have not been able to do for a while, things like going horseback riding, canoeing, skiing, or riding a roller coaster? Pick some things that you have not been able to do since you gained weight and use them as your motivation. There is a good chance that your weight gain has limited you in some way, with regards to things that you enjoy doing (assuming you were not always overweight). Let's use them as your motivation to lose weight.
- Do you want to make a good first impression? Being thinner and fitter always helps you make a better first impression for both business and personal relationships.

Another set of important questions to ask are:
- What is your biggest fear in life?
- Do you think that losing weight and getting fit might reduce or eliminate this fear?
  - Is your biggest fear death? Could you live longer if you were at a lower weight?
  - Is your biggest fear your finances? What would health problems do to your finances?
  - Is your biggest fear being bedridden? Do you think that losing weight and getting in shape will help you stay healthier?

25

- Is your biggest fear not finding a job or losing your job? Do you think that losing weight and getting fitter would enhance your appearance to your customers, prospects, management, or future employers? Would it give you more self-esteem, increased energy, and a better attitude?

Whatever your greatest fear in life is, losing weight and getting fitter can probably help ease that fear. Let your fear be a motivator.

I have posed a lot of questions and challenged you to really take a good look at yourself. These are the same questions that I ask myself on a daily basis to serve as a reminder of my goal and to keep me on track. Look back to these questions frequently throughout your weight-loss journey when you need affirmation that you have made a health commitment that will make your life better.

Understanding what makes you do something is important, because if you can learn to deal with those factors differently, you will be on the road to losing weight.

What Makes You Overeat

Stress is one of the biggest reasons people gain weight.

These days most people are stressed. People are losing their houses, their retirements, and their jobs. What is there not to be stressed about? What you may not know is that stress actually causes your metabolism to slow down. If you eat in order to deal with your problems, you have the recipe for weight gain. That is because you are using food as a distraction from the problems of life.

When you eat, it makes you feel good. You feel satisfied. The feeling that food gives is calming and relaxing. It fills an immediate need, and it gives you a feeling of control. The problem is that you gain weight. This weight gain adds to your stress, which makes you even more stressed out. What happens next is that you eat even more, and the cycle goes on.

There are a few things that you can do to reduce stress. The first is to change your thinking about your stressors. Stress is not caused by the actual event but by your thoughts in reaction to the event. This is hard to do, but if you can change how you internalize your stress, you can reduce it.

As you work on changing your thinking, there are strategies you can also use to reduce stress on your body.

- **Exercise**
  One of the best ways to reduce stress is to exercise regularly. This always works for me. Always check with your doctor before starting any exercise program. Even before the weight loss, when I was stressed out about something I would exercise a couple of days in a row. It really helped me relax. I believe that exercising is a better release for stress than eating. It gives you time for yourself, which allows you to think and address the problems that are facing you. It also allows you to blow off steam. When you are done exercising you feel better, you are more relaxed, the stress is

lessened or gone, and you are in an improved frame of mind. This is just what you need when you are stressed out.

- **Foods**
Stress on the body can be increased by what you eat and drink. Sugar, salt, some fats, and caffeine have an adverse effect on the body and therefore should be reduced especially when you are feeling stressed.

- **Antioxidants**
Eating and drinking foods high in antioxidants (e.g. acai, blueberries, cranberries, raspberries, pecans, and many more) give your body and brain what they need to run optimally. This can help counteract the effects that stress has on your body.

- **Breathing**
Has anyone ever told you to take a deep breath when you are stressed out? There is a reason for that. When you take deep breaths and then release them slowly, more oxygen goes into the body and more carbon dioxide is released. This helps the body reduce stress.

Deep-breathing Exercises

Deep-breathing exercises are a good part of a weight-loss and exercise program. The benefits include:
- Weight loss
- Stress reduction
- Increase in immune system functions
- Relaxation
- Release of tension
- Increased movement of toxins out of your body via the lymphatic system

Deep-breathing exercises are easy to do and can be done just about anywhere. Also, it doesn't take much time to do it. The hardest part is just remembering to do it daily. Check with your doctor if you have any respiratory problems or other concerns.

There are many deep-breathing exercises out there. However, the one I like is:

Breathing Exercise

Do this while sitting down. Stop if you feel light-headed or have other unpleasant side effects.

1) Count from 1 to 6 while taking a deep, slow breath and breathe in all the way.

2) Hold your breath while counting from 1 to 8. (It's ok if you can't go the entire time at first.)

3) Breathe out while counting from 1 to 7.

4) Repeat 6 times, or less if needed.

If you add breathing exercises to your daily routine it can help reduce stress levels, support your weight, give you a better attitude, and give you better health. The hardest part is just remembering to do it.

- **Massage**
  A good massage can help reduce muscle tension and stress on the body.

Once again, I am not a doctor and this section is not meant to be a biology lesson, but to let you know that stress can cause you to gain weight if you are not careful. The bottom line is that it is important to manage your stress if you want to manage your weight and there are strategies that can assist you.

Boredom is another reason for weight gain.

Some people eat when they are bored. When you eat, it gives you something to do when you're bored, helps pass the time, and leaves you physically satisfied. I recommend exercising instead when you are bored. It will pass the time away, it won't cost you money for food, and you'll feel good and relaxed afterward. If boredom causes you to eat in the evening, find a hobby to occupy your time so that you don't have time to snack. Plan your evenings so that you don't get bored. Have a list of projects that can keep you busy so that you don't eat. Find things to do that burn calories.

The answer is simple: If you are a boredom eater, don't let yourself get bored.

People gain weight when their routine changes.

Some people gain weight when their schedule or routine changes. This is what happened to me. I went from being single, an employee at a large auto supplier and having a set routine to having a wife who is a good cook, running my own computer company and having no set routine. This is when the weight started to come on.

When I started running my business, I was home a lot. My office was next to the kitchen. This was a bad combination. Then as my business grew, I found myself out at lunch time, and I would go to the local fast-food restaurants for lunch. This was the start of a very destructive habit. This habit which not only cost me a lot of money was also leading me down a road of weight gain and potentially future health problems, a road I unknowingly did not want to go.

If your job keeps you on the road, the answer is simple: pack a healthy light lunch. If you work from home, keep yourself so busy that you don't get bored and attack the refrigerator constantly. This takes planning the night before so that you have productive tasks to occupy your time, which in turn won't let the boredom cause you to eat. Even with your head in the right place, old habits and thoughts can still creep in. Just remember, it probably took years to develop the thinking that got you overweight. It will take three to six months to get thinking right, but could take many years to keep the wrong thinking from coming back. Incorrect thoughts about food and exercise will consistently test your commitment. This is known as temptation. However, on a good note, as time goes on temptation will occur fewer times in between. You will enjoy being thin, you won't want to be overweight again, and food will have a lesser meaning to you.

People gain weight when they fall in love.

Do you ever notice that people who get into relationships tend to put on weight? Why is that? There are a couple of reasons I see. The first reason is you tend to eat out more when you are dating. The combination of eating out and drinking more tends to pack on the pounds. My suggestion here is to pay very close attention to what you order when you go out. Although you may have been scolded by your parents for not cleaning your plate as a child, as an adult you don't have to lick your plate clean. You can leave food on it. Also, relationships tend to upset routines and habits which, as we saw above, can cause you to gain weight.

Whatever the emotion, eating satisfies a short-term need, and that is the problem. The issue, the reason, the stress or the boredom doesn't go away. Once again, if you are a stress or boredom eater, try exercising. It is a fantastic way to work off stress, nerves, anxiety and boredom. Whatever your reason for your overeating and snacking, find an alternate and long-term solution.

You will also need to develop a delayed gratification mindset so that you can get the long-term rewards. If you start every day with a focused plan and focused commitment, you will be able to avoid these types of destructive eating.

Another part of understanding why you are overweight is to understand your beliefs and attitudes. The next section will discuss how your beliefs and attitudes about losing weight will determine your weight-loss success.

Your beliefs and attitudes play a big role.

Do you believe that you have a choice about whether you are thin and fit? Do you believe that your weight problems are the consequences of your bad choices or the result of uncontrollable circumstances? The answers to these questions show your beliefs about your weight and can explain why you have a weight problem.

Where do your beliefs come from, you may ask? They come from your history and your current environment. They come from your parents, your friends, your boss, and your co-workers. They even come from what you have read in the paper, heard on the radio, saw on the internet, and watched on TV. All of these things helped form what you believe about the control you have over your weight. Sometimes these beliefs about your weight and your ability to lose weight are inaccurate, but they all had a piece in forming your core beliefs about weight, health, and fitness.

These beliefs are what formed your attitudes and your emotions about losing weight and getting fit. Your beliefs can create intense, negative emotions. These attitudes create the excuses you use and contribute to self-denial. These strong emotions drive your actions and your inactions which over time become your results (i.e. overweight / obesity).

You need to understand where your beliefs came from and then find a way to deal with them. An example of this is, "Well, I am heavy because it runs in my family. It is genetics." In this example, this person was told growing up that she will be overweight because many in her family are overweight. The problem is that person actually became overweight because she adopted her family's bad eating habits, not because of her genetics.

Your beliefs on how you view weight loss, health, and fitness will determine your success or your failure in losing weight and getting fit. Do you associate weight loss with starvation, eating bad foods, and having to give up your favorite foods? Do you feel that good health is something that you have little control over? Do you think that if you don't think about it, then you won't have health problems? Lastly, do you associate exercise and fitness with a lot of hard work and pain? If you answered yes to any of these questions, is it any wonder why you can't lose weight or keep it off? It is not fun for you, the process is painstaking, and so you avoid it. You procrastinate and never get to it. These beliefs have to change if you are going to lose weight and keep it off. You will need to enjoy the process and focus on the results to win the battle of the bulge. For instance, if you don't like to exercise you won't do it for very long. However, if you get yourself to enjoy exercising then there is a good chance you will do it for the long term. Jogging is hard. Jogging is a lot of work, but I enjoy it. I found an exercise that I enjoy and that I will stick with. Find an exercise you will enjoy doing. Find two or three and rotate them so that you don't get bored.

Are you a person who doesn't want to give up overeating and fattening foods? If you change your thinking, this can also be enjoyable. It is all how you look at it. Since I don't overeat anymore, I don't feel sluggish, tired, or bloated after meals. I have not stopped eating my favorite foods, although I have definitely cut back on the quantity I eat. How is this enjoyable, you may ask? You change your attitudes towards food. First of all, you want to get the attitude of eating to live, not living to eat. This one was and is the hardest for me because at my core, I love to cook and love to eat. My attitude has changed tremendously by trying a variety of foods and preparing the foods differently.

As you start to lose weight, something will happen. You will look at food and start to ask yourself, "Is this worth eating?" You will then realize that overeating and eating fattening foods only gives you short-term gratification, but also long-term discomfort, stress, and a shorter painful future.

If you think that the process will be torture, it will be. Your thinking, which generates your attitudes, will determine the outcome. If you think the process will be fun, you can make it that way. It is all how you look at things. I have found that there is one of two pains that overweight or obese people must endure. These are the pains of change and regret. The key is to make change a fun challenge so that it can actually be enjoyable and painless. It is all about what you decide to focus on. Are you going to harp on the negatives or get excited about the positives? Your attitude, which is how you react to things, will determine your success or your failure. Your attitude and your emotions is your thinking in action.

Belief that you can lose weight is a big accomplishment. A business mentor of mine once told me that there will only be action if the belief is there. You must have the belief that you can lose weight. I will go even further and say that you must have 100% belief that you can lose weight. If you only have 80% belief that you can do it, the other 20% will find a way to stop you in your tracks through obstacles, adversities, and self-doubt.

Just remember that I am not exceptional, and I did it. Furthermore, you are not so exceptional that you can't do it. In other words, if I can do it anyone can. You can do it if you have the desire, the belief, the commitment, and a plan. Your attitudes and beliefs towards losing weight and getting fit are more important than the obstacles you have in your life keeping you from it. Your attitudes will determine your failure or success, and your *Reason Why* will keep you driven.

The next step in the process is to take responsibility for where you are (your true current reality) and to take responsibility for losing the weight (where you will be in the future).

Step 3
Take Total Responsibility

"Remember the three R's:

Respect for self.

Respect for others.

Responsibility for all your actions."

Unknown Author

Before you can lose weight you have to accept responsibility for your weight and for your fitness. What does this mean? It means that you are in control over your weight and your fitness. This means that you can do something about it. You cannot control the weather, you cannot control the economy, you cannot control whether you will have a job tomorrow, but you can control what, when, and how much food you put in your mouth. You can control if, when, and how much exercise you get, and you can control how you spend your free time. You control your schedule, and you are the only one responsible for your weight and your fitness.

One of the first things you need to do is to identify all your excuses for not losing weight and getting fit, then work on eliminating all your reasons and excuses why you can't. It just takes one excuse to keep most people from losing weight. Start telling yourself, "There will be no more excuses." Take control of your future or your bad health will do it for you. In case you didn't get this important concept, let me say it again in a different way. Make the right changes (lose weight) before your health forces you to.

When people initially saw that I lost a lot of weight, the most popular question they would ask was, "How did you do it?" No matter what I told them, they almost always responded the same way. They would say that they wanted to lose weight but…excuses … excuses... excuses, blame... blame… blame.

People use excuses to justify, quite frankly, their immaturity. I was immature with respect to my weight, and if you are overweight you probably are too. My kids use excuses daily to justify their poor actions and bad decisions. That is nothing short of immaturity. We as adults are immature when we make excuses for our poor actions and decisions with respect to eating and exercising. It is all about maturity, and we need to take responsibility for our weight, health, and fitness if we want to be mature adults. Once again, I will be the first to admit that I was immature with respect to my weight. However, I did something about it. Are you willing to do something about it?

If you decide not to exercise, aren't you deciding that being fit is not important? If you decide not to watch what you eat, and how much you eat, aren't you deciding that losing weight is not important? Whether you realize it or not, you are making that decision. That is the bottom line.

If you say to yourself that you are mature about your weight, then you need to make the right decisions and take responsibility for those decisions, and you need to do something about it. The not-so-pretty alternative is to remain immature and overweight, and to blame everyone and everything for your poor decisions. Either way, it is your health that will be affected, no one else's.

The lack of taking responsibility and showing immaturity (when it comes to our weight) shows itself in the form of excuses. So I am going to start by giving my definition of an excuse.

My definition of an excuse is, *"A lame reason to justify a poor decision to yourself and others."* Remember that doing nothing is a decision.

I have another story to illustrate this point. After I lost 40 of the 50 pounds, I went to the doctor for my yearly physical. My doctor congratulated me for my results and asked me how I did it. I explained to him that it was the change in my thinking that allowed me to make the changes needed to lose weight. My doctor then told me about a patient he just saw. He mentioned to this guy that he really needed to lose weight. This guy's response was, *"I can't lose weight because my wife puts too much food on my plate."* This guy needs a good smack on the back of his head for that excuse. After thinking about it, I realized I was there a couple of years ago, and you may be also.

"People are always blaming their circumstances for what they are. I don't believe in circumstances. The people who get on in this world are the people who get up and look for the circumstances they want, and if they can't find them, they make them."

George Bernard Shaw

In other words, people who are successful in losing weight don't make excuses, and they don't play the blame game.

Let's discuss some of the more popular excuses I hear daily for not losing weight. If you are using one of these excuses, stop it immediately. Challenge your excuses and let them go.

"It's all in the letting go."

Shirley Garrett

Excuse 1: "I do not have time."

If I gave you and your family a week vacation to Hawaii, unless of course you live in Hawaii, there is a good chance that I would not be able to get you on the plane fast enough. You would probably cancel everything you had planned that week and go. You would spend the time to plan your itinerary, have time to pack, and have time to go shopping. Now, if I ask you to exercise regularly, you use the excuse that you don't have the time? That is because it is not that you don't have the time. It is that you choose to spend that time elsewhere, and that is because exercise is not important to you. However, if you say that your health is important but your actions speak differently, what is that saying? Once again you are in denial that since you happen to be fine right at this moment, it is not important. In reality, this is the time to get the weight down and get fitter. Once you lose your health, it is hard and painful to get it back, if you can get it back.

I hear this excuse every day from people. They don't have time for their health, but they sure have time for watching reality shows. They don't have time for their health, but they sure have time to watch sports. I remember making these same comments. I used to think this way also. But once again excuses are really nothing short of immaturity. What is maturity? Isn't it choosing what you need to do over what you want to do? You can always find the time for things you want to do. You just have to want to exercise, and it has to be important to you. Then and only then will you find the time.

The best way to do this is to concentrate on the results. Keep your eye on the prize which is your *Reason Why*. DO NOT, I repeat, DO NOT focus on the process. Focus on the results, and you will figure out how to fit exercise into your schedule. For example, why not ride an exercise bike, walk on a treadmill or use an elliptical machine while watching your favorite TV shows? Use your TV time as a workout time as well.

Make it a priority and make it happen. Once we put importance on it, we will carve out the time in our schedule to get some exercise in. Like they say, "Where there's a will there's a way."

I am married, I have two small children, I own multiple businesses, and belong to a couple of organizations, yet I make time to work out. How, you may ask? I will tell you.

I made it my # 1 priority for four months.

It took priority over just about everything, including my family. I came to the conclusion that if my health declined, or worse, if I died of a heart attack or a stroke, it would have a devastating impact on my family and beyond. So I made my health, my weight, and my fitness my #1 priority for four months. I realized that my health is the foundation for everything in my life.

Now that I am thin and fit, I am able to ease off some. I still exercise regularly, I monitor my weight daily, and I am ready at any time to move health and fitness back to the #1 priority for a day or two to get my weight back on track.

If you are too busy after work to exercise, get up a half hour to an hour earlier to exercise, or exercise during your lunch break by going for a walk. It is a choice and you are responsible for making the time, whether it is before work, after work, or during lunch. You are in control.

You are in control of your time, and you are also in control of whether you allow other people to waste your time.

Excuse 2: "I'm too tired."

That is the very reason for losing weight. If you lose weight and get fit, you will feel better and have more energy. I have also found that if you can push yourself to work out when you are tired, it will reinvigorate you, and it actually releases the stresses of the day. If it is easier, you can get up an hour earlier and exercise before work.

Excuse 3: "Weight problems run in my family."

If the excuse you like to use is that being overweight is genetic, I want you to know that my father was very overweight, and I managed to lose weight. I did so because it is my choice and my responsibility how much food I put in my mouth, what I put in my mouth, and how much I exercise.

The tendency to become overweight may be genetic, but if you develop the right thinking you can change that. I have another theory. Instead of the cause of your weight struggle being genetics, maybe it is nothing but bad eating habits being passed down from generation to generation. Who fed you when you were younger? Your parents did. Therefore, you developed your eating habits from them. If they had poor eating habits, they probably taught them to you. They set the bad example that you then picked up and kept. What you need to do is to break that cycle.

I chose to break that cycle. I chose to put less food in my mouth. I chose to put some healthier food in my mouth, and I choose to exercise regularly. As a result I lost 50 pounds, and since I did that, I am not moving in the direction my father did.

I actually got to see the cycle of learned behavior in action first-hand. My youngest son eats fruits and vegetables. He will pick a fruit salad over fries. He will pick a piece of fruit over chips most of the time because we had them in the house when he was younger.

When my oldest son started eating solid foods, we did not have fruits and vegetables in the house for him to try. Therefore, he does not like them, and we are still today struggling with it. This illustrates that it is all about setting the example. Bad eating habits by kids are acquired from their parents. Remember that your actions are more powerful than your genes.

Excuse 4: "I watch what I eat but I still can't lose weight."

"Never mistake motion for action."

Ernest Hemingway

This excuse I hear a lot from people: They think they are eating healthy and/or exercising but can't lose weight. If you are in this situation you may be feeling hopeless. There are things you can do.

Maybe you just need to start keeping track of what you are eating and how much you are eating.

If you are eating healthy but still cannot lose weight, you may want to try adjusting your portion sizes. That should resolve the issue. Beware that healthy foods can contain a lot of calories.

Later in the book I will be discussing the importance of weighing yourself daily. The reality is that you may be losing weight all week and gaining it back with one or two days of indiscretions.

Albert Einstein said, *"Insanity is doing the same thing and expecting different results."* If you want to lose weight, and you are not, then you need to do things differently.

If what you are doing is not working, don't get mad. Don't get upset. Just change what you are doing. Different results will only come with different actions.

I am not big on counting calories. However, I have learned through my ups and downs what foods put weight on me and what foods don't. And I have learned how much of certain foods I can eat and how it affects my weight.

This is important, so listen carefully.

I was asked if I always eat healthy foods all the time. The answer is no. What has kept me thin is the fact I sometimes eat what I want but in smaller portions. This allows me to feel that I am not depriving myself of anything. Therefore, there is nothing to stray from (i.e. a diet) as long as I control my portion size.

It is all about balance. It is balancing the foods that I love with healthy foods to maintain a good weight.

Excuse 5: "I don't want to give up my beer."

Once again, *"Insanity is doing the same thing and expecting different results."* If you want to lose weight you will have to change some things. You will have to cut back (not give up) to lose weight. I am not saying to give up your favorite foods or drinks. What I am saying is to cut back, so that you can occasionally enjoy the things you like and still lose weight. This is not a good excuse.

Excuse 6: "I travel much in my job, and have to stay in hotels and eat at restaurants."

This excuse was told to me the first time by a very large man. First of all, most hotels have workout rooms and/or pools. Secondly, there are usually healthy, low-calorie choices on the menu to pick from at restaurants. No one said it would be easy, but it can be done.

Excuse 7: "I have a slow metabolism."

This is a good excuse. This excuse is one that you don't think can be verified. Well, it can. I saw a news report a while ago that took a group of women who thought that they could not lose weight because of their metabolism. They sent the women to a doctor to test them. It was found that all of these women's metabolisms were normal for their age. They were totally shocked of course and embarrassed into admitting that they needed to do something different. If you noticed I said, "for their age." As we get older our metabolism does slow down; that is a fact. What this means is that our bodies require less food to maintain our weight. With that being said, should we eat like we did at 18 years old? The answer is absolutely not! If our bodies require less food to operate, we need to learn to give our bodies less food. Also, exercise has been proven to increase a person's metabolism. So, for all of you who use the metabolism excuse, start exercising and eat less.

Excuse 8: "My job requires a lot from me."

I hear all the time that my job requires too much from me. That is just another excuse for not taking responsibility for your weight, health, and fitness. Your work can't control your free time.

I will also let you in on a secret. Exercise is a great stress reliever. Exercise is better than food for releasing stress. Exercise gives you the time to think about the issues in your life and your work, and because you will be more relaxed after your workout, solutions seem to come easier. Moreover, most jobs don't require you to eat lots of fattening foods, so you can always pack a healthier, lighter lunch.

Excuse 9: "It is the fast-food restaurants' fault."

If you are one of the people that blame the fast-food industry for your weight problem, I just have one thing to say. Stop it. It is not their fault. You made the choice to eat there, and you made the effort to drive there. This does not make you a bad person, but on the other hand, you need to take responsibility for those bad choices you made in the past, and you need to move forward into a better and healthier future.

I feel that fast-food restaurants provide a valuable service. If you are overweight you need to pass on that service or make better choices when you go there. Do not blame them for your bad choices.

If you are caught out and are forced to go, then do what I do. Order one item from the dollar menu. Even though it may not be the healthiest thing for you, the portion is usually small and it won't affect your weight much if at all. You don't need to order a large meal and triple-size it.

Excuse 10: "I have to leave my office at lunch to get a break."

I used to go out to lunch every day. A guy who sat next to me talked me into going out for lunch. His reasoning was that he needed to get out of the office for an hour. If you need to get out of the office at lunch, just grab an apple, go for a walk, and get some fresh air. That will clear your head better than sitting in a fast-food restaurant. You will also come back to work revived and with an improved attitude.

Excuse 11: "I have tried many diets and none of them worked."

"Never, never, never, never give up."

Winston Churchill

Many of life's failures are men who did not realize how close they were to success when they gave up."

Thomas Edison

The problem is that you are dieting. The answer to that is not to diet. Diets are something you go off of and gain the weight back, sometimes with interest. Develop a plan that you can live with forever. When you diet you usually give up a lot of the things you love. The thing is that you can strategically have those things. You just can't eat those things all the time and not in high quantity. For instance, I love potato chips and ice cream. I don't eat them as often as I used to anymore. When I do, I have just a small pinch of chips, not an entire bag (never sit with the bag of chips - you will eat the entire thing) or one scoop of ice cream. The hardest thing for most people to accept is that there is no easy way to lose weight. I have not seen a diet that tells you to sit on the couch, eat anything and everything you want, and you will lose weight. Losing weight is simple but not easy.

The first three letters in the word diet make up the word *die.* Why is that? That is because you will kill yourself trying to stay on it long-term.

What has happened in the past will not happen in the future if you don't let it. What matters is what you do now. This is a fresh start. Today is the start of your future, and what you do with it is your choice.

Excuse 12: "Big is Beautiful"

There is a saying that "Big is Beautiful." As I looked in the mirror and saw my three chins and my big belly, I wondered what was beautiful about it. Yes, you can be beautiful on the inside and big on the outside. Here's a different thought: How about being beautiful on the outside and inside? How about being the best person inside and outside you can be? I think sayings like this give people an excuse for doing absolutely nothing about their weight and health. I think it promotes a cavalier attitude about being heavy and unhealthy. What they are actually saying is that it doesn't matter if you are heading for diabetes, high blood pressure, and other health problems as long as you are beautiful on the inside. They are even saying that you may die young, but people will say you are beautiful on the inside.

If I just raised your blood pressure, great. Our society today has really made it acceptable not to take any responsibility for any of our decisions. This attitude concerning your weight and health can kill you prematurely. Some of you are saying, "Well George, I have tried to lose weight and failed many times." My answer to that is, GREAT, now you know what doesn't work. Let's try again.

Big is not healthy, high blood pressure is not healthy, and lying in the hospital room hooked up to machines is probably not going to look beautiful. So, let's not glorify being overweight - let's do something about it.

47

More on Excuses

Before you can lose weight and keep it off, you must first have control over your mind, your thoughts, your choices, and your habits. You must be in control of yourself. You must know your true reality (true reality being where you are, not the rosy glasses you view yourself with), and you must take responsibility for where you are and where you want to be.

You might be saying, "Well George, you don't know my situation. I am different, I have a special situation."

Whatever you think, you're not so special that you can't lose weight. If your schedule is too full, then empty it. Are your kids in many sports? Cut back on some. It is your choice how you spend your time.

If health issues are keeping you from exercising, talk to your doctor to see what you can do.

I will repeat this again because it is very important. First you need to take responsibility for your weight and for your fitness because no one else is going to do it for you. Quit making excuses and quit blaming everything and everyone. You are responsible. If you want to be fat then admit it, continue to do nothing about it, and move on. Don't try to justify your actions by making excuses and blaming everything and everyone you can. You are responsible. It is your body. What you put into your mouth is your choice, and how much you exercise is a choice. If you have been doing this, it does not mean that you are a bad person. It just means that you need to realize what you have been doing, and you need to stop doing it.

The Bottom Line
Most of us like to blame our special circumstances as our reasons or excuses not to do something. We like to look for someone or something to blame when, in reality, our problem is how we see things and not our current circumstances.

The bottom line is that your excuses will stop you from losing weight. They will even keep you from starting the process.

So let's challenge all your excuses. Remember that doing nothing about your weight only hurts you and your family's future.

After you see your true reality, find your ***Reason Why***, take responsibility for where you are and where you want to be, and challenge your excuses, it is time for action. It is time for results. The time is now. You can win the battle of losing weight and keeping it off. It starts with one single good decision, and continues with another good decision after another. Like the old Chinese proverb says, "A journey of a thousand miles starts with a single step."

It is important to take constant daily steps towards your weight loss and fitness goals to achieve success.

The list on the next page shows the results of using excuses for not losing weight and also the results for developing reasons for losing weight (followed by action). You will notice that they both will give you results. However, excuses will probably give you the results you don't want. If you want good results, it will require some changes. We will examine change more closely in the next section, and how it can be good or bad.

The list below illustrates two points:
1) What **excuses** for not losing weight can result in.
2) What **reasons** for losing weight can result in (if followed by actions).

Excuses Can Result In

Overweight, Obesity
Poor Health, Sickness
High Blood Pressure
High Cholesterol, Cancer
Diabetes, Heart Attack
Pills, Shots, Stroke, Death
Immobility, Hospitals
Pain, Sorrow, Loss, Grief
Financial Ruin
Lost Relationships

Reasons Can Result In

Being Thinner, Fitter, Longer Life
Good Health, Mobility
Lower Blood Pressure, Good Appearance
Higher Energy
Success

Change Can Be Good or Bad

If you want to change your body, if you want to change your fitness, if you want to change your health, you need to change your thinking and what you are doing. The bottom line is that you have to change.

Change can be hard, but only if you think it is. Change can be work. For a flower to grow and for a flower to bloom, it has to change. For babies to grow to adults, they must change.

Throughout life your body changes, and with that change, you need to change the types and quantity of foods you eat. If you use the excuse that your metabolism is the reason for your weight gain, then it is logical that you should eat differently now that your body has new requirements.

Most people just need one reason to keep themselves from losing weight. All it usually takes is one excuse to keep people from starting. Don't give yourself one.

Who are you hurting if you don't start? You are not hurting me! You are hurting your friends who will have to watch you destroy yourself! You are hurting your co-workers who will probably have to pick up your slack! You are definitely hurting yourself and your family. You are hurting your future and the future of your family. Think about that.

If I had a car and didn't get oil changes and tune-ups regularly, the car wouldn't run well and would eventually fall apart over time. It would not happen overnight, but in time the car's engine would be destroyed. The same thing happens with your body. If you think any different you are in denial. If you don't care, then what you are telling everyone is that you don't care about yourself, and you don't care enough about your family to do something about it.

Since you are reading this book I assume that you want to take action. The next step is to set a goal and then take action on it.

Step 4
Set a Goal & Take Action

Good Intentions

"The desire to do something doesn't get it done."

Unknown Author

"Action may not always bring happiness, but there is no happiness without action."

Benjamin Disraeli

You cannot lose weight by just having good intentions. You need to take action. Wanting to lose weight is not enough. Telling yourself you want to lose weight won't work. Once again, I refer to Albert Einstein's words, *"Insanity is doing the same thing and expecting different results."* If you want to change your weight, then something must change in what you are doing and what you are thinking.

If you want to go from 200 pounds to 160 pounds then there is only one course of action: burn up more calories than you take in. That's it. It is that easy, yet that complex.

Every day you make choices. Exercise or sit on the couch and watch TV. Eat a light lunch or go out for lunch and double-size your meal. Whatever choices you make will either take you towards your weight goal or move you farther from that goal.

I have come up with an equation that further explains this:

$I * A = R$

This stands for:

Intention * Action = Results

The formula works this way. If you have good intentions about losing weight but do nothing about it, you get Zero results.

Good Intention * 0 = 0

In the example above:
(You want to lose weight) * (You don't exercise and change your eating habits) = Your weight does not change

Let's look at the next example:

If you have good intentions and do the opposite action, you get negative results. An example of this would be having good intentions to lose weight then going out for fast food every day. If you are trying to lose weight, but you end up gaining it, you are doing negative action (i.e. not exercising, overeating, and/or eating the wrong foods).

I was at a restaurant for a business meeting. A young obese person with me ordered a 20-ounce cut of prime rib dinner. This person ate the entire thing, ate the potatoes, left the salad, and then ate the ranch dressing that came with the salad using a spoon. A week later this person told me about having to get knee replacements. I asked this person if he thought losing a little weight would help the knee problems. He answered that it probably would not matter. He then told me that he was actively trying to lose weight. See this person's reality. He eats a 20-ounce piece of prime rib, eats the baked potato with all the toppings, drinks the ranch dressing without the salad, and that is the way to lose weight? Sadly, that is the reality most of us have. Good intentions are great but without actions it is meaningless. In this person's case, it is more like negative action, which will give negative results (weight gain).

Good Intention * -Action = -Results

In the above example:
(You want to lose weight) * (eat a 20-oz prime rib / potatoes / drinks) =
Weight Gain

If you are asking why the multiplication sign instead of an addition
sign, the answer is simple. There is a multiplying effect that goes along
with the action, hence the multiplication sign. The higher and more
intense the action is, the more explosive the results.

Daily actions toward your weight goal must be taken, or you will get no
results. Remember that good intentions, no matter how good, without
taking action to support them, are only a dream.

"A goal without a plan is just a wish."

Antoine de Saint-Exupery

We also need to understand and remember that focused daily actions
are the only things that matter.

The next step is to set a goal and then create a plan.

Set a Goal

"The future that we study and plan for begins today."

Chester O. Ficher

What exactly is a goal? A goal is a destination toward which you direct resources like time, energy, and focus. I am convinced that the only obstacle standing between you and your weight goal is the commitment to stay determined and focused. Let's have the insight to know you are not where you want to be and have the belief and commitment to know you can get to your weight loss and fitness goal.

A goal is specific. A goal is measurable. A goal is an accomplishment. A goal also needs to be completed within a specific timeframe and will include resource constraints. For example, how much time are you willing to dedicate for exercising? Can you afford a gym membership? Are you willing to take the time to track your weight? Without setting a specific goal, your weight loss is nothing but wishful thinking. So, you need to make sure that you know what you want before you start.

When I first told a business associate of mine that I was determined to lose weight, he immediately asked me two questions. How much weight are you going to lose? By what date are you going to lose that weight? I was initially taken aback by those two questions but thought for a moment and gave him an answer. I then realized what he was doing. He was asking me about my goal. A goal has to have a start date, end date, and a desired weight. How else are you going to know if you are successful? This is very important. I picked my son's birthday as my goal date, which meant that my initial goal was to lose 30 pounds in just under two and a half months. I hit my goal two days before his birthday, and then I set another goal. I am not telling you this to brag but to show the power of a clearly defined goal. Setting a goal forced me to make the right choices daily, so that I could hit that goal. I also picked an important date: my son's birthday. We were planning a pool party for the family. I actually wanted to look good for the party. In reality, it didn't matter because my family knew I was overweight, but it was something I could latch onto. It was my extra motivation. A goal will help you see your future self and allow you to chase it.

Let's go through the process of setting a goal and applying action to it:
1) Currently, what is your weight?
2) What weight do you want to be?
3) When are you going to start (how about now)?
4) What is the date you want to be that weight?
5) What are you going to do to hit this goal?
6) Chart your weight daily.
7) Keep daily track of your food and exercise.
8) Review your results and adjust as necessary.

This will be discussed in more detail in the following section.

Here are few very important things about goal setting:
1) Put your weight and fitness goals in writing and post them where you will constantly see them.
2) Be specific when defining your goal (exact weight and date you will reach it).
3) Define the maximum time and resources you are willing to give to achieve this goal.
    a. How much effort will it have taken you when you say "you're done"?
    b. Looking at your time and resource constraints will force you to place a value on losing weight, which will force you to prioritize less important things.
4) Visualize your goal daily.
5) Make your goal achievable.
6) Set a timeline for the goal.
7) Break the goal into manageable parts.
    a. What will your weight need to be next week to hit your goal?
    b. What will your weight need to be in two weeks (etc.)?
8) What obstacles are you going to incur?
9) Plan for, remove, or minimize obstacles ahead of time.
10) Review progress daily.
11) Give yourself a reward for hitting the goal (not a big fattening dinner).

Remember that a non-serious person will say, "I am trying to lose weight." A really serious and dedicated person will say, "I will lose _____ pounds (you pick the pounds) by ___/__/____" (you pick a date). Which are you?

Do you see the difference? When you say that you are "trying" to lose weight, it means you really are not going to. Trying gives you a way out. Well, I "tried" to lose weight but… excuse….excuse….excuse….

Have you ever invited someone somewhere and that person said that he or she would "try to make it" and then didn't? It is a nice way of saying, "I won't be there." It is the same way with losing weight. Don't try to lose weight, DO IT! There is no time like the present.

A Chinese proverb says, "A journey of a thousand miles starts with but a single step." This means that to get thinner and fitter, you need to do the hardest task: you need to *START*. It also means that the action of starting will take you on the road to results.

Goal Sheet for Losing Weight

Your current weight: _____

Your goal weight: _____

When are you going to start (now is a good time)? _____

What date will you lose the weight by? _____

What is your core reason for losing weight (Your Reason Why)?

_____

_____

What are you willing to do to get to this weight? (This shows your commitment level.)

_____

_____

Is there a specific area you want to concentrate on? _____

What actions are you going to take in the next 12 hours towards the above weight-loss goal? (This shows you are serious.)

_____

_____

Create Checkpoints along the Way

Let's say you want to lose 30 pounds in three months. That is 2.5 pounds per week. If you weigh 200 pounds and want to be at 170 pounds in three months, then you need to create a chart like the one below.

If you start the fitness journey on May 1 and by August 1 you need to be at 170 pounds:

Date	Your Weight	Goal Weight
May 1	200	
May 7	196	197.50
May 14	193	195
May 21	191	192.50
May 28	191	190
Etc…...		

In the above example, this person did not always hit his weekly goal. I did this on purpose because there were weeks that I did not hit my goal, while other weeks I passed my goal. Obstacles, setbacks, and tests of your commitment WILL happen. It is part of the process for losing weight. Don't let it get you down. A little later in the book I will talk a bit about obstacles and setbacks and how to deal with them. Remember to set a goal, write down a strategy, and follow it.

I recommend breaking down a larger goal into smaller ones, because on the weeks you do well, that will fire you up. However, on the weeks you don't do well, you can use it as a learning tool to see where you went astray, and to see what you need to change.

Another thing happens when you break your goal down into smaller pieces. It becomes more attainable than this big goal, far into the future. Furthermore, it doesn't leave you hanging at the end. You will always know where you stand. Like I said before, there are times you are going to overshoot your goal and times you are going to miss your goal for the week. However, you are going to learn from those experiences, and you will learn what works and what doesn't. The key is to learn how your body works. There is nothing that will give you more satisfaction than hitting one of your smaller weekly goals, and nothing better to give you the confidence that you can do it.

There are three other items you must have to be successful. In addition to a goal, you must have commitment, determination, and focus.

Commitment, Determination, and Focus

"Do or don't do; there is no try."

Yoda

"Few things are impossible to diligence. Great works are performed not by strength, but by perseverance."

Samuel Johnson

As I asked earlier in the book, have you ever said or heard someone say, "I am trying to lose weight..." or "I tried to lose weight but ...?" What they are really doing is showing a lack of commitment. Some may call this lip service. It is like asking people to do something, and they say they will "try" to do it or "try" to make it. Experience tells me that they usually don't.

One of the things I realized was that my health is my most important asset, and I need to set it as my number-one priority. This is because I realized that without good health nothing else matters. People say *time* is their most important asset; other people say money is their most important asset. However, in reality, it is your health. If you have your health you can always make more money. If you have your health you can live longer and have more time. So, good health should be your most important asset. How are you taking care of that asset? Are you abusing your body or are you investing time and energy into it so that you have good health? Are you investing the time and energy for your future?

To lose weight you need to have three things. You need to have an intense commitment, determination, and you need to stay focused. You need to commit to your weight-loss goal, you need to make a commitment to yourself, and you need to stay focused. You also need to have the determination to follow it through to completion. Once again, your commitment, determination, and focus need to be intense, constant, and long-term, which is the very reason you need a strong enough **Reason Why**.

When I was in the groove of losing weight, I was intensely determined and committed. People told me I was a fanatic; people told me I was obsessed. That is how I knew that I was in the groove. From the outside, intense commitment and determination looks like obsession. Remember that the end game is to have better health, so don't do anything that is unhealthy (like skipping meals or not eating).

If you truly have intense commitment, determination, and focus, action will follow. If you procrastinate and push off your goals, your frustration will increase. Procrastination also means that you don't have the drive, the motivation, and a strong enough **Reason Why**. Set a weight and fitness goal, commit to it, and get started. My three questions to you are: What is your goal? When are you going to commit to it? What initial step are you going to take today?

"It's always too soon to quit."

Norman Vincent Peale

Every action and inaction will move you towards your weight-loss goal or move you away from it. Next, I will list a few positive actions you can take to move you towards your goal, along with some negative actions you should avoid.

What Actions Will Help You Hit Your Weight Loss & Fitness Goals?

- Exercise a minimum of four days a week.
- If you are forced because of circumstances to go to a fast-food restaurant, order one item from the dollar menu. (The portions are small.)
- Do something active after dinner.
- Eat two pieces of fruit or a small salad for lunch.
- Have a maximum of two alcoholic drinks a week.
- Reduce or eliminate sugary sodas and foods.
- Weigh yourself daily.

What Actions Will Take Away from Your Weight Loss & Fitness Goals?

- Going out for breakfast or lunch more than once a week.
- Going up for seconds at mealtime.
- Overfilling your dinner plate.
- Sitting on the couch after dinner for the rest of the night.
- Eating three big meals in one day.
- Eating a bag of chips for a snack.
- Having a drink or two most days after work.
- Overindulging-eating or drinking too much.
- Blaming others.
- Making excuses.
- Letting your emotions control you.
  - Using food to make you happy or lift your spirits.
  - Eating when bored.
  - Eating when depressed.
  - Eating when stressed.

Fill out the Weight-Loss Action Form to assist you with your weight-loss plan.

Weight-Loss Action Form

What **actions** you are going to take: Goal Date:

1._____   1._____
_____

2._____   2._____
_____

3._____   3._____
_____

4._____   4._____

Projected Results:

Immediate Goals (2 weeks):

Long-Term Goals:

What obstacles / constraints do you anticipate?

How are you going to overcome the above obstacles / constraints?

Cost: (What resources are you willing to give, such as time, money, and commitment?)

Which one of these actions can you take today to move towards your goals of losing weight and getting fitter? If the hardest thing to do is to start, which of these actions can you start today? Let's start the process by referring to our *Reason Why* and showing your commitment by taking the first steps towards a thinner and healthier future.

Meals

If you are like I was, you probably love certain foods, and you likely have bad eating habits which keep you from losing weight. What most people do is try to give them up altogether. They give up their fast-food, their chips, their ice cream, or their chocolates. But for most people giving up the foods they love is a weight-loss disaster waiting to happen.

That's why I am going to show you how to incorporate the foods you love and still lose the pounds you desire.

If you ever planned a vacation, you know that it is important to know where you are going to stay, how you are going to get there, how long it will take you to get there, and what you are going to see when you get there. Losing weight is the same way.

To lose weight you need to know where you are, where you are going, how you are going to get there, and how long it will take you to get there. You also need checkpoints along the way so that you can verify that you are going in the right direction and are on schedule. If not, you need to change direction and/or speed.

Below are samples of the steps that need to be taken to succeed in losing weight:
1) Create a weight-loss plan.
2) Commit and do the plan.
3) Measure your progress.
4) Revise your plan and start over at #1.

The first thing is that you need a plan, a plan that works for you. A plan you can live with. This plan will be the start of a lifestyle change. It doesn't have to be complex, but you need to have one, and it starts with your meals.

Below is a similar plan I used for my meals. It gives you a good indication of what I did to lose weight. However, you don't have to use this plan. Remember that every person's body is different, with different caloric needs. The object is for you to create a plan that works for you. Create a plan that you can live with from this point forward.

George's Meal Plan
- **Breakfast (pick 1)**
  - 2 eggs, using only 1 yoke, fried with non-stick, no-calorie spray
  - Yogurt
  - Cottage cheese and fruit
  - Non-sugary cereal w/low fat milk

- **Lunch (pick 1)**
  - A meal replacement bar
  - A protein bar
  - A large apple
  - 2 bananas
  - Yogurt
  - Cottage cheese and fruit

- **4 o'clock Snack (pick 1)**
  - 1 small fistful of peanuts
  - 1 small fistful of sunflower seeds
  - A small fistful of raisins

- **Dinner**
  - Anything you want (with these rules)
    - No seconds or thirds
    - Cut your usual first portion by a third to a half

- **After-Dinner Snack (pick 1)**
  - Small bowl of grapes
  - A banana
  - An apple
  - 5 wheat crackers with block cheese
  - 1 fistful of trail mix
  - A *pinch* of chips (not a bag)
  - 1 small scoop of ice cream

If you look at the above meals you will see that I eat two small, healthier meals for breakfast and lunch as a general rule. The 4 o'clock snack is there to cut my hunger before dinner. As for dinner, I have what I want, without overdoing it. And for a snack I rotate healthy and non-healthy snacks. At the beginning, I had a hard time giving up my ice cream and chips. I knew that totally giving them up would result in failure. Instead I opted to include them in my plan, but on a limited basis and in small portions. This gave me the feeling that I was not giving anything up. As I started to lose weight, I got excited and opted for the better choices on the list.

Again, this plan allows me to *balance* the foods I love with healthier foods so that I don't feel deprived. If I don't feel deprived there is nothing to stray away from because there was nothing I went on (i.e. a diet). If I want something, I eat it for dinner but in a smaller portion.

If you are saying to yourself, "Well George, I can't do this. I would starve," you are most likely eating way too much food and need to train your body to eat less. That's of course if you are really truthful about the reasons you want to lose weight. The concept of losing weight and creating a new lifestyle is simple. No one said it would be easy, but it is worth it.

> *"Insanity is doing the same thing and expecting different results."*
>
> *Albert Einstein*

It is all about self-perception. I had to restructure the way I ate, the things I ate, and the amount I ate to obtain my goal. I also had to be mentally okay with it and look at it positively, not as a chore, not as a painstaking task. To do that I incorporated things I like to eat into my plan, even though they were not the healthiest for me. It is not about giving up all the things you like to eat. It is about moderation, it is about balance, it is about a core lifestyle change. Most people will never give up the things they love to eat, but they can cut back. They can eat those things in moderation.

Live a life of moderation. You can start by eating more fruits and vegetables. Then cut your lunch and dinner down by a third to a half (and no seconds). Make sure you eat at least three times a day. The five tiny meals a day work better and help to speed up your metabolism.

The next plan you will need to create is an exercise plan.

Exercise Program

"Push yourself: No pressure, no diamonds."

Mary Chase

First of all, always remember to consult your doctor before starting any exercise program.

Exercise can be fun if you make a game out of it. Pick an exercise that you will enjoy and that you are willing to do for 45 minutes, four to five days a week. There are many to choose from, such as walking, running, biking, swimming, elliptical machine, treadmill, aerobics, yoga, rowing, cycling, martial arts, etc. Is it easy? The answer is no. It can be hard exercising when you don't feel like it. Like the quote above says, "No pressure, no diamonds." Goals take work. They take action, but it can be enjoyable, especially when you start to see results. Remember that the more work, the greater the commitment, the faster you get results.

You can also add other exercises like taking the stairs, which is a great way to burn calories. If you like watching television, exercise while you are watching it. This is a good way to fit some exercise into your schedule and not miss your favorite shows. You can walk or bike when it makes sense. If you are the person who fights for a front spot in parking lots, stop doing that. You can burn calories by parking in the far end of the lot and walking.

It is a good idea to look at your dream, dread, or **Reason Why** and figure how much time it will take to get there. For example, my son plays the electric guitar. He needs to make time for his lessons, and he needs to make time every day to practice.

No matter what, you must be committed, determined, and focused on your goal, so you can get to your destination.

When I started on my new journey of weight loss and fitness, I started running three days a week. My legs really could not handle any more days of abuse than that. As the weight started coming off, I increased the number of days I ran, the distance, and the time. I was able in a short time to get up to a six-mile run six to seven days a week. Now, you may be saying that is too much abuse on your body no matter how much you weigh. I will agree with that. I just kept that schedule until I hit my goal. I did this until I went into the maintenance mode. Then I cut back to three to four days of running a week.

I did this for one reason: momentum. There are two ways to lose weight: fast or slow. I prefer fast. The faster you lose weight the more motivation you will get because the results are coming fast. Some people think that losing weight slowly will be less painful. What occurs is that they rarely do lose the weight they want to lose. This is because they are not in the battle. It is not on their minds constantly. Therefore, they make poor choices, and as a result, they don't lose weight.

Exercising regularly can lower blood pressure, cholesterol, and blood sugar and help in a variety of cardiovascular ways. It can even make you look younger by toning muscles and sculpting your body.

I don't want to spend a lot of time here on exercising because there are lots of great books, videos, and websites on the subject. Keep in mind one thing: The exercising you do can be simple, and you don't have to join a club, but you do need to have the commitment to it. You need to start, and you need to do it consistently. If you don't, you may pay for that decision down the line.

Step 5
The Daily Weight-Loss Process &
Using the Scale

Have Fun and Enjoy the Process

If you are like most people, you may think that to lose weight you have to figure out how much weight you want to lose, figure out what it will cost you, and then pay the price. That is how you lose weight. Having this train of thought will lead to failure. That is because who wants to do anything painful? Who wants to pay the price?

The idea is to make the process fun so that there is little or no price to pay. Yes, you will have to invest time, energy, and hard work. However, it is an investment in your future, not a drain on your time and energy. You will also need to learn some new habits and unlearn some old ones as part of the process. This can be both different and exciting if you want to make it that way. It is all up to you.

Losing weight and getting fit is what you make of it. If you can find a way to make the creation of a healthier lifestyle fun, you will have a better chance of succeeding.

If you look for the fun in it, you will find it. If you look at the work you will be undertaking, you won't last. The results are dependent upon your perspective. Make exercise fun, not a chore. Look at food differently. Look at eating big lunches as making you tired and bloated in the afternoon. Look at changing some of the food you eat as an adventure in trying new foods. Just have fun, enjoy the process, and enjoy the journey.

Monitor Your Weight Daily

One of the best tools in your weight-loss toolbox is your scale. Therefore, if you don't have one, get one. (I prefer a digital scale because I feel they are a lot easier to read.)

Conventional weight-loss wisdom says that you should weigh yourself once a week. This is so that you see the results of the week, and you can measure those results weekly. I totally disagree with this. You must weigh yourself daily. Not only should you weigh yourself daily, you must weigh yourself at the same time daily. The best time to do it, I have found, is in the morning. I have made it a habit to get up, go to the bathroom (hope that's not too much information), then weigh myself. One of the reasons why I lost fifty pounds in four months and have been able to keep it off is because I monitor my weight daily. I make sure that my weight doesn't go up a pound at a time and catch me off-guard. See, as I have mentioned, losing weight is about the daily choices that you make. How do you monitor those daily choices? You weigh yourself daily. If you weigh yourself daily you will see how well you did the day before. Did you exercise or not? How did that affect your weight? Did you eat too much of this or that? What is the scale saying? Should you have eaten this and this? What did the scale say? It is your daily report card. It tells you if you made the right choices the day before.

Let's say you are doing what you need to be doing all week and actually are losing weight. Then that one day during that week you overdo it, ruining the entire week's work. If you weighed yourself weekly you would probably quit and say that you can't do it, it does not work, etc... Now let's say that you weigh yourself daily. You see the weight coming off during the week, and you see that bad day in the form of a weight spike. Your attitude will be different. You will see what happened and analyze the situation and adjust for the next time. You will see that your plan is actually working, but that you are human and messed up.

The scale helps keep you honest, gives you a daily reality check, tells you if you are doing a good job or not, and allows you to see the results of your daily choices. There were times that I knew I messed up the day before and gained weight. When (not if) this happens to you, it is still very important to step on the scale. It is a hard thing to do, and it is difficult to admit to yourself that you screwed up. It is easy to skip weighing yourself that day. You need to weigh yourself anyway. It will allow you to admit to yourself that you made a mistake, and it will definitely make you feel guilty, which will allow you to make better choices that day and in the future.

One thing I want to acknowledge is that a woman's weight can vary naturally throughout the month. It is possible that a woman will not see a direct correlation between actions and her weight during certain times of the month. If a woman identifies those patterns overtime, she will get to know her body even better.

Monitor your weight daily, track the results, then review your results, and make the correct adjustments. **Remember to make it a habit to do it every day at the same time**. The preferable time is in the morning right after you get up, and then follow the daily process I have outlined on the next page.

The Daily Process

I have a simple and quick daily process that I still use even today to not only lose but maintain my weight.

1) **Weigh yourself**
    Check your weight (first thing every day). You need to know where you are so you know if you have results.

2) **Make a plan for the day**
    Develop a plan for the day. It does not need to be a long, drawn-out plan. You just need to take a few seconds and come up with a quick plan for the day. This will allow you to accomplish your goal for the day. If you want to lose weight, what will you eat for breakfast today? What will you have for lunch? How much will you eat at dinner? When and how long will you exercise today? What healthy snack will you eat instead of ice cream or chips? If your weight is where you want it to be then put a plan together for that, and have the ice cream. It is all about planning.

3) **Execute the plan for the day**
    Do what you say you are going to do. You need to keep the commitment you made to yourself in the morning.

4) **Check the results (weigh yourself the next day)**
    The next day you need to check your results by stepping on the scale. Ask yourself these three quick questions:
    a. Am I at the weight I want to be?
    b. How did I do compared to yesterday's weigh-in?
    c. What did I do yesterday that caused my weight to go down, go up, or remain the same?

5) **You may or may not need to make some adjustments**
    Depending on your results, reflect on what you did right, what you did wrong, and what you could have done better.

6) **Repeat 1 through 5**

If you are maintaining your weight, your plan will be different because you can just keep doing what you are currently doing. If your weight goes up a couple of pounds, spring back into the weight-loss plan for a day or two until your weight goes back down.

If you repeat this process daily, and you stick to and execute your plan, you will lose weight. I still today execute this plan daily to monitor and maintain my weight and to keep my weight in check.

That is the daily process I used to lose weight and maintain it. It is that simple. However, the hardest part is just starting. Remember the Chinese proverb that states, "A journey of a thousand miles starts with a single step." So for this to be effective, you must start. You must take that first step. You must make the first good choice, and continue to make one right choice after another. If you mess up, you are only one good choice from getting back on the right road. You are human, and you will mess up. I sure did. Even today I occasionally still mess up. My mistakes are becoming fewer and farther between, but it still happens. However, I immediately get back on track because I weigh myself daily, so that I can catch it and deal with it swiftly.

See, your mind will continually test your resolve. Your mind will deceive you if you let your guard down. It will tell you that you did okay the day before when you didn't, but the scale will always tell you the truth and keep you honest. That is why your scale is the most important tool, your best weapon, in your weight-loss battle and in maintaining your weight, your health, and your fitness. You need to treat it that way, so that you can develop a very good habit of weighing yourself every morning, from which you can create a habit of putting together a plan, executing the plan, checking it, making course-correcting adjustments, and doing it again.

It is about balance. I give myself a five-pound swing. If I hit my upper limit, I watch how much I eat and what I eat, and I exercise more for a day or two. If I am at the lower part of the range, I can indulge myself a little more.

However, as a rule I have a light breakfast and light lunch, and eat what I want for dinner. I just watch the quantities at dinner. Having what I want for dinner allows me to feel that I am not giving anything up. Therefore, there is no diet to go off of. It is very important to never skip a meal. That could actually give you the opposite results you expect. When you skip a meal it tells your body to store fat. This of course is not a good thing.

I want to end this section by stressing once again that you need to weigh yourself every day. I still weigh myself daily to keep my head in the game, and to keep myself on the right road.

Step 6
Take the Right Road

I truly believe that **anyone** can lose weight and keep it off, but like I always say, "You must first win the battle of the mind before you can win the battle of the bulge."

You must first change your thinking before you can change your body. You must change your thinking about food, exercise, health, and fitness. Only after doing this can you change your weight for the long haul, which will take you on the right road to a longer and healthier future. It is important to be aware that until your thinking changes, you will not be able to change your results.

If I ask you what comes to mind when I mention the words "losing weight," would you say discipline, starvation, having to give up your favorite foods, having to eat bad and tasteless foods?

If I ask you what comes to mind when I mention the word "exercise," would you think of pain, sweat, exhaustion?

If "losing weight" and "exercise" means those negative things to you, it is no wonder that you have not been able to lose weight. Look at it this way: Since I have changed the way I eat, I have more energy, I am not tired after I eat, I feel better, and I look younger. Furthermore, I have come to realize that I enjoy being thin, and that I like how thin looks and feels more than I like to eat. Consequently, I would rather be thinner than go up for seconds or thirds.

Exercise needs to be fun. You have to enjoy it; you have to want to do it. Only then will you do it. I enjoy it. A long run relaxes me. It gets rid of the stress of the day. It is my time. It allows me to think and solve problems. The best thing is that I like how it tones me up. It bothers me if I have to miss a workout. Only when you enjoy it will you do it long-term.

The key is to take control of your thinking so that you can take control of your weight, fitness, and health, and you need to look at exercise as something positive and not negative. You need to concentrate on the positives of the results and not the negatives of the process.

If you look at the weight-loss and fitness process as negative, you won't do it. It is natural for people to avoid things they don't like or don't want to do. We as people don't usually do things that are uncomfortable or cause us anxiety. If you look at weight loss and fitness as negative, guess what, you won't do it long-term, if at all.

How do I look at things? I look at exercise as positive. I love to exercise. Exercise gives me more energy. It causes me to lose weight so I feel better. Exercise tones me up. Exercise makes me look younger and it helps clear my mind. Exercise relieves the stresses in my life. When I exercise in the morning, it gets my blood going, I feel great all day, and it gives me a better attitude. It keeps me relaxed so that things don't bother me as much. When I exercise at night it relieves all the stresses of the day. If I come home exhausted, exercise revives me and gives me my second wind, helps me clear my mind and work through the problems of the day, and helps me to be creative. Given the two attitudes, one that loves to exercise, and the other that hates it, or views it as a necessary evil, which attitude has the best chance of exercising long-term, and which attitude will eventually quit or not even start?

My History with Food

I want to let you know where I came from concerning food, so that you can see how I had to change my thinking. First of all, I love food. I live to eat, not eat to live. When I was younger I learned how to cook my favorite meals so that I would never have to go without them or depend on anyone to cook for me. How could I lose fifty pounds? I had to change my thinking. Do I still love food? You bet. However, I had put together an eating system that works for me so that I didn't feel deprived.

What did I learn? First of all, I had to realize that I am not young anymore and cannot eat anything I want in massive quantities. Then I learned that although I eat three meals a day, only one is a serious meal. The other two are light meals, a small bowl of cereal in the morning, or two eggs or even a yogurt and a piece of fruit. For lunch I eat a large apple or a protein bar. I always eat something light, and I don't skip any meals. I was not a big fruit or vegetable eater. I was a meat and potatoes kind of guy, but I found fruit I learned to enjoy, and the more I ate it the more I enjoyed it.

Then about a half-hour before dinner I learned to eat a fistful of peanuts or sunflower seeds. The idea here is to help spoil my dinner so I don't pig out. I eat what I want for dinner, just a reasonable portion, and I don't take seconds or thirds. I don't deprive myself of anything. If I want a greasy burger, I eat one. Do I make that burger a pound? I do not. This allows me to feel that I have not deprived myself of anything. I did not go on a diet. Therefore, there was nothing to go off of. I just changed my lifestyle of food and exercise to a lifestyle of balance.

When I was in my teens, I remember going to a restaurant with my parents, ordering two meals and polishing it off with a banana split, and I did not gain a pound. However, now that I am older I cannot eat that way. I accepted that, and I changed my mindset.

Since I started eating lighter, I noticed a few things. When I ate a huge breakfast or lunch, it actually zapped my energy. When I ate a big breakfast, I felt terrible. The food felt like a lump in my stomach. After a large lunch, I would want to take a nap. Now, I eat a piece of fruit or two for lunch, and I don't feel tired. As a matter of fact it even gives me more energy. I also feel more creative, I have a better attitude, and I am more productive throughout the day.

You need to change your thinking and attitude towards food and exercise, and turn it into something positive, so that you will want to do it and get positive results.

If you agree how positive it is eating light meals for breakfast and lunch as opposed to larger meals, then it will be easier for you to make that transition to smaller meals. If you find the positives instead of the negatives you will be on the right road, and you will succeed.

In Step 2 I talked about having a *Reason Why*. You will need to concentrate on your *Reason Why*, so that you can focus on what you want, not on the process.

A good example of this is going on a vacation. When you go on vacation do you concentrate on all the things you will get behind on?

Do you concentrate on the time you have to spend packing, all the shopping you will need to do? Do you concentrate on the money you will be spending? Do you concentrate on the long car ride? Do focus on the hassle of flying? If you focused on all those things you probably would not go. What you concentrate on is relaxing and sitting on the beach. You concentrate on how much fun you will have, because all the rest is the process of what you have to do to get there.

It is the same way with losing weight. You need to concentrate on what it is going to be like when you are thinner and not the process. Yes, you have to go through the process, but you don't have to concentrate on it. The fact is that when you are thinner you will have more energy, be able to get in and out of the car easier, climb those stairs without huffing and puffing, and find that the pain in your back and legs are reduced or gone because the weight is not beating on them. So once again, concentrate on the end game not on the process, because if you concentrate too much on the process you won't even get started. If you concentrate on what you want and back it up with actions, you will be on the right road to a longer and healthier future.

Whether you know it or not, you are traveling down a road concerning your health. The question you need to ask yourself is, "Which road am I on?" Are you on the road to a long and healthy life where you are fully active in your 80s and 90s, or are you on the road that will lead you off the cliff to a heart attack or stroke? It is your choice. The road you are traveling on is determined by the choices you make every day. Where you will be tomorrow is determined by the choices you make today. You make these choices every day, whether you think about them or not.

Some of the choices you make include:
- Do you exercise today or not?
- Do you bring a small, healthy lunch to work or do you go out for fast-food?
- Do you grab those chips or grab an apple?
- Do you go up for seconds or not?
- Do you go up for thirds or not?
- Do you grab an unhealthy snack or a healthy one?
- Do you walk up the stairs or take the elevator?

- Do you park in the back of the parking lot to get more exercise or fight for a close parking spot?
- Do you sit on the couch after dinner and vegetate or do something to burn calories?
- Do you make excuses for your weight or find reasons to lose it?
- Do you make excuses for why you cannot lose weight or look for new things to try?
- Do you concentrate on the results or focus on what you are giving up?
- Do you take vitamins daily or skip them frequently?

Many of these decisions are made in a split second. The choices you make will determine which road you are on, and those choices will determine your future. Good or bad, they will determine your future. Sometimes even the little choices add up and become amplified over time, which can have major consequences down the line. Furthermore, every choice either keeps you on the right road or takes you in a different direction. Keep in mind that doing nothing is a choice.

I often see that people don't make the connection between the choices they make (which many times they don't even realize they're making) and their consequences. Every choice you make has a ramification that can change your future for better or worse.

I tell my kids all the time that their choices have consequences. I tell them that good choices have good consequences and bad choices have bad consequences. The interesting thing is that they don't always see those consequences, and they don't always want to admit that the consequences will affect them. That is because the consequences are not always immediate. It is the same way with your weight and that is why it is so important to see where the current road you are on is taking you, and where your choices are taking you.

What are the ramifications of your lack of exercise? What are the ramifications of your past, current, and future eating habits? Are you choosing to trade instant gratification for long-term health consequences? It all starts with one choice, and therefore, we can get on the road at any time with just the first right choice.

Although you can get back on the right road with just the first right choice, how difficult is it to get your health back once you start having health problems? The time to get on the right road is before you have major health issues, not after you get them. You may find it is difficult to fix your health once it goes bad. Start making the right choices today and get on the road to better health.

In a commercial I saw the other day, a woman said, "I am too busy to have a heart attack." Although on the surface the commercial was humorous, it was also sad and true. I see people all the time wait until something happens to them before they do something about their weight. By that time, it is too late. The damage has already been done.

The "If it ain't broke, don't fix it" attitude does not work with respect to your body because once it breaks it will cost you time, money, and pain. Furthermore, in the end you may not be able to fix what you broke because of your poor choices. The answer is not to let it get to that point. You need to make the right choices sooner, not later. Therefore, if you are too busy to have a heart attack or a stroke, then take a little time to get thinner and fitter so you won't have to give a lot of time later.

You need to start thinking about every choice that you make, at least at the beginning, until this becomes a habit. As a side note, a good habit usually takes 20-30 days to form. However, the temptation to revert back to your old bad habits can be there for years.

The reason you don't think about the bad choices you make is because they have become a habit. If you start making the right choices, over time they will become good habits, and in time you won't have to think about them anymore.

The key is to start thinking about every choice you make and ask yourself, is what you're about to do moving you towards your weight goal or away from it.

I want to talk about the two roads of weight loss. The first road will lead you to a longer and healthier life. The other road will lead you to health issues. The first one takes some time and effort up front but pays off in the future. The second one takes no time, and no effort now, but can cost much pain, time, effort, and money in the future.

Given a choice of these two roads, take the first one. It will actually be easier later and will be worth it. Would you rather put in a little effort now, which is something that you can control, or would you prefer to wait until your health goes, at which point it controls you? If you want to stay in control of your life, start by controlling your weight. If you don't, you will lose that control because your poor health will control you. Getting on the right road is not easy; changing directions can be difficult, but it is definitely worth it.

As Einstein said, *"Insanity is doing the same thing and expecting different results."* If you want different results in losing weight, you need to do something differently than you are doing now or your results won't change! You need to make changes in your life if you want to change your life.

Think about it. How you think about food and exercise got you to where you are today. If you don't like the view in the mirror, things need to change. There is no magic pill, and no quick fix that will get you thin and fit. Change your thinking, change your attitude and change the road you are on to a better future.

I know of no guarantees in life that ensure if you do all the correct things, you will have a long, healthy life. There is a very high probability that if you are not on the right road, your future won't be a healthy one.

In reality, there is no risk for losing weight and getting fit, but you risk your future if you don't. If you don't want to do it for yourself, then do it for your family and friends. It is never too late to start.

I have two stories that illustrate two different people on very different roads. The first person is on a right road, with a long and healthy future; the second person is on the wrong road heading for the cliff.

The person on the right road:
The other day I had a meeting with a person I grew up with. This guy has been thin all of his life, and recently I found out why. When I got

to his house, I realized that he forgot about our meeting because I woke him up. While I was there he had breakfast. It was an orange and a banana. I was impressed but didn't say anything at that time. Later, he got a call during which he made dinner plans to meet people at a pizzeria. I realized he had developed a balanced eating habit, which worked for him. It was the same habit I developed. He was careful and ate light and healthfully for breakfast and lunch, which allowed him to indulge at dinner. He had that lifestyle his entire life. The great part of it was that it was a lifestyle that worked for him. He is on the right road, and it showed. He embraced this and it worked for him. It worked for him, it worked for me, and it can work for you. Later, I talked to him about his eating habits and he verified exactly what I just told you. He stayed thin by eating a light breakfast, a light lunch, and whatever he wants for dinner, without overdoing the portion. Balance is one of the keys to weight loss.

Now for the person on the wrong road:
I recently meet a 30-year-old man who was obese. He told me he takes medication for high blood pressure and is a diabetic. I asked him if he thought that he could eliminate these pills and shots if he lost weight. He said probably, but didn't sound interested. He is an example of a time bomb ready to explode. This man is in denial and is on a shaky road with a questionable future in sight, and it was sad to see.

Years ago I was on the wrong road. My weight was going up every year, and I was in denial about it. As a matter of fact, I too wasn't even aware I was on the wrong road. However, after I had my *Ah-Ha Moment* and after I found my **Reason Why**, all of that changed. I made one decision. One decision followed by good choices, and that got me on the right road.

If you are at Point A (which is where you are today), and you want to go to Point B (a long and healthy life), there is only one road. Anything else is the wrong road that leads towards the cliff. If you are on the wrong road it is time to turn back. It is time to get a map, which is your reality check, and get on the right road by making the right choices.

There are two choices. Either make the commitment to travel on the right road to a healthy weight or make the decision not to do so. The choice is yours along with the consequences.

The choice is also yours as to whether you make this journey hard or easy, because it is all in how you look at it. It is all in your thinking.

Think the right thoughts, make the right choices, and do the right actions. Making a lifestyle choice can be tough, but it definitely is not impossible. It will take commitment, it will take focus, it will take determination, and it will take a different way of looking at things. However, it can be done, and it will be worth it.

 I truly believe that you can travel on the right road and become thinner if you choose to be, but only if you are willing to change your thinking and follow it with the right actions. Just remember the old saying, *"Nothing ventured, nothing gained."*

Step 7
Overcome Obstacles

I want to start this section off with a sailing story. A few years ago after a beautiful sail, I was heading down the Detroit River to dock my boat at the marina. I went to start my engine and guess what? It would not start. I kept trying and trying, but the engine would not start. So a buddy of mine who was sailing with me asked me what I was going to do. I told him we were going to sail into the well. He laughed because he knew that it was going to be a challenge. He knew I would have to gauge the wind and the current so that I stopped the boat exactly where I needed to. However, what he didn't realize was that I sat in the back of my boat many times planning for such a problem and going over different scenarios. I had already done it in my head. I didn't have to come up with a solution under duress because I knew what I needed to do. I had already overcome that obstacle. Problems are inevitable when you have a boat, and so it was a matter of time before it happened. Therefore, I prepared for that day so that when it did happen, I knew exactly what I was going to do, and it ended well.

The same idea can be used for losing weight. Obstacles and setbacks will always occur. It is just part of the process. As long as you stay focused on results, you can overcome them. You have the ability to get thinner and fitter but a lot of times losing weight looks like too large of an obstacle. If you want to lose weight and get fitter, you have to learn to see these obstacles differently. You need to prepare for the obstacles that will throw you off the road you want to be on. I had many obstacles come my way. One obstacle was boredom eating. I ate when I was bored. I would attack the snacks with a vengeance. I also ate when I was stressed. I had to overcome pigging out at buffets and parties. When there was that much food I would go crazy. I encountered many obstacles I had to learn to overcome.

Overcoming your obstacles is a very important part of changing your thinking so that you can lose weight. It is mandatory that you learn to deal with these obstacles so that you can lose weight because the obstacles are not going to go away; the key is to learn how to deal with them.

How do you deal with these obstacles along with others you may face? The answer is to deal with each one separately. First you need to know what drives you to eat. Then you can deal with them one by one.

For instance, let's look at boredom eating. Like I said earlier when I was bored, I would attack the snacks with a vengeance, whether I was hungry or not. How did I learn to deal with that? I make sure I never get bored. I have a list of things I want to accomplish, small thing and large, easy things and complicated, and when I get bored, I attack the list instead of the snacks. I keep myself busy.

How did I handle stress? I used to eat. Now when I am stressed I exercise. I have found that exercise allows me time to work through what has stressed me out. I can play it over and over and over in my head and when I am done exercising, I am relaxed, at peace, and I have a different perspective. Exercising allows me to find solutions to problems because it gives me focused, uninterrupted time to think. When I am stressed usually I have some anxiety and excess energy that exercise also helps eliminate. It sure beats eating and sitting on the couch, where nothing gets resolved and I gain weight.

One of my biggest obstacles was buffets and parties. When there is that much food I used to go crazy. I have come up with a few things to help me through them. Before I get in line at a buffet, I walk the buffet to see what is there. That way instead of taking everything, I only take the things I really, really want. In other words, I take my number one items. Sometimes I take the salad plate and use that instead of the large dinner plate, so that I can limit my portion easily. It is also a good idea to sit as far away from the buffet table as possible so that it is an effort to go for seconds. Furthermore, I try not to face the buffet so that I am not staring at it. I also like to use the 20-minute rule: If you want to go up for seconds, wait 20 minutes before you go. I have found that I rarely want to go up for seconds. Those are strategies I use when I go to a party or an event with a buffet.

Another obstacle I had to overcome was overeating when my favorite foods are put in front of me. I just could not stop eating them. What I do now is after food is made, I take enough for one reasonable meal and freeze the rest before I sit down for dinner. Make sure to divide the food into small portions so that you can eat it more often, but not in large enough quantities to damage your weight. I have found that this works really well for me. This also allows me to have the foods that I want because they are there all the time, but packaged in such small portions it doesn't affect my weight.

The last obstacle that I want to talk about is emotional eating (sadness, excitement, etc.). In the case of negative emotions, food made me feel good. It gave me instant gratification. In the case of strong positive emotions, it was the fact that I didn't know what to do with the emotions. Eating in this case helped calm me down and gave me something to do at that moment. Once again, I found that most extra eating can be stopped by either exercising or by just finding productive things to do to stay busy.

You will have obstacles. This is not an if, but a when. They are part of the process. If you did not have any obstacles in your way, you would already be thin. Those obstacles have kept you where you are. You will also continue to have them until you change your thinking and learn how to deal with those obstacles.

"Adversity causes some men to break, others to break records."

William Ward

Most people stop when they hit a roadblock. They stop when they hit an obstacle. They say, "I can't do this. I cannot go any further." However, the person who overcomes the obstacles is the one who wins, the one who loses weight.

What you also need to do is to focus on your **Reason Why**. If you have lost weight and gained it back, or have not been able to lose weight, it is only because you haven't found a powerful enough **Reason Why**. I am going to say this again, because it is very important. It is all about focusing on what you want, not on the process or the problems. When you change your focus to what you want, you will overcome your obstacles.

It's like going on vacation. Let's say you're in the car heading down the road, and you run across a construction detour. You wouldn't stop and say, "Well, I am going to turn around and go home. This vacation stuff is just too much for me. I am never going to get there. This is extremely hard." You get out a map or GPS and find an alternate route, or you follow the signs to get around the obstacle. That is because you are motivated to get to your destination. You are focused on the destination. You don't focus on the problem; you focus on getting around the problem.

It is the same with losing weight. Focus on what is important, not on the little stuff. Obstacles are just small things that get in your way and keep you from accomplishing what you want to accomplish. The bad part is that this is where most people get stopped. They get stopped on these little obstacles instead of going over them, through them, or around them. Don't let this happen to you.

Whatever your obstacles are, identify them and plan for them because they will happen. Plan what you are going to do when they happen just like the sailing story I told earlier. Plan what you are going to do when you go somewhere that has a buffet. Plan what you are going to do at the next party. Plan what you are going to do when you are bored, and then keep going over it, and over it, and over it again, so that when faced with those obstacles you are not making emotional decisions (oh, the food looks so good). You are making smarter decisions. That is because you already conquered it in your head.

Identify your obstacles, plan for them, and eliminate them.

Step 8
Develop the 7 Attitudes
of a Thin Person

How Do You Know When Your Thinking Is Right?

I am always asked this one specific question: How do know when you are there? How do you know when your thinking has changed? The answer is simple. Eventually, good thinking and different attitudes result in better decisions and actions which over time develop into the right habits. A habit is something you do on a regular basis, and that you really don't have to think about. Therefore, when you develop a certain set of good attitudes and habits, then your thinking has changed. I am going to discuss what those attitudes and habits are so that as they start to occur you will realize that your thinking is actually changing. Never become complacent. It is easy for your old thinking to return. It will constantly test you. The tests will happen small and slowly, without you realizing it. It starts off innocent. It only takes one day of indiscretion without a correction day (a day that gets you back on track). You say to yourself, well it is only a pound or two. A week later it happens again, and you start moving off the right road.

Attitude #1: Thin people rarely overeat or binge.

The first attitude is that thin people rarely overeat or binge. This includes piling up food on your plate. It also includes going up for seconds, and thirds. Thin people rarely overeat. See, if you make the decision not to exercise, overeat, and eat the wrong foods, you are making the decision to be at an unhealthy weight, but if you make the decision to exercise, eat healthier, and eat smaller portions, you are making the decision to be thinner and healthier. It is the decisions you make daily, that determine which road you are on.

This is how I think about overeating these days. When I overeat it is like having a lump in my stomach. Overeating is uncomfortable. If I have a huge lunch, I usually want to go back to the office and take a nap. Don't you? If I have a big breakfast I feel sluggish all morning. If I overeat at dinner I usually want to sit on the couch and vegetate the rest of the night. If I overeat before I go to bed, I have a restless night.

Overeating is uncomfortable. Overeating really zaps my energy level. So why would I want to do it, and why would you want to do it?

Sometimes you don't plan to overeat, it just happens. You eat and eat and eat, then about a half hour later it hits you. To avoid this I use the 20-minute rule. I take a reasonable portion of food and eat it, I wait 20 minutes, and if I am still hungry I will take a little more. If I am not hungry, I am done. Almost every time I find that I am not hungry and therefore won't eat any more. That keeps me thin and it can also keep you from overeating.

If you want to be thinner you have to train yourself that less is better. You have to develop the mindset that bulging at the seams does not feel good, so that you won't want to do it. If you want to be thinner and stay that way, you have to stay away from overeating and binging.

Attitude #2: Thin people exercise regularly.
The second attitude of a thin person is that they exercise regularly. To exercise routinely you have to enjoy the process of exercising. If you want to become thinner you need to find exercises that you enjoy doing. Whether it is walking, jogging, or bike-riding, you need to find something that you enjoy doing, and something that your body can handle. Your doctor is a great resource for helping you select the right exercise. As always, consult your doctor before starting any exercise program. Exercise will help you lose weight, get fit, become healthier, and give you a good attitude and a better frame of mind, but the process has to be enjoyable or you won't do it long term. If you want to be thinner and fitter, you need to know that exercise is important. You need to like to exercise because of the results you get from it. You need to look forward to exercising and feel guilty if you have to skip a workout. If you want to be thinner and stay that way, you need to exercise regularly.

Attitude #3: Thin people take responsibility.
The third attitude of a thin person is that they take responsibility for what they put in their mouths, they take responsibility for their exercise, and they also take responsibility for their health. What does this mean to you? You need to know that you are in total control. It's about taking control of your body, taking control of the choices you

make daily. It is not making the easy choices but the right choices. The easy choice is going out for lunch and triple-sizing. The right choice is having an apple and going for a walk. It is sometimes making the tough mature choices. However, once you see the results it will fuel your motivation. It will pump you up, give you confidence, and give you faith that you can do it, which will push you to make more of the right choices.

After I lost my first 25 pounds I was really excited, and it gave me the confidence that I could do it. It showed me that I could take total control of my body. It is about the choices you make. It is about knowing that **YOU** can choose to be overweight, or **YOU** can choose to be thin, and that it is your choice. It is your responsibility. One of the reasons you are overweight besides not having a strong enough *Reason Why* is that you have not decided to take responsibility for your weight, health, and fitness. It is about maturity (with respect to your weight). Mature people take responsibility for their daily choices, and for many years I was immature when it came to how I treated my body, how I ate, and my lack of exercise. You need to take responsibility and make the right choices as a mature adult, and you need to make these choices into a habit so that you don't have to think about them.

If you want to become thinner and stay that way, you need to take responsibility for your weight, fitness, and health. You cannot make excuses, you cannot blame anything or anyone for where you are, and you need to do what needs to be done, because you are responsible and in control of your decisions.

Attitude #4: Thin people choose the right snacks.
The forth attitude of a thin person is that they choose healthy snacks the majority of the time. I am not saying that you always have to choose an apple over chips, but what I am saying is that if you want to be thinner and stay that way, you will have to pick healthier snacks the majority of the time. Can you eat that candy bar, those chips, that ice cream? Yes, you can, but you cannot eat them all the time and not at the same time. The majority of the time you need to make healthier snack choices if you want to be thinner.

Attitude #5: Thin people don't diet.

The fifth attitude of a thin person is that they don't diet. You don't diet, you change your lifestyle. You develop a lifestyle of balance. You balance the things that you love with healthy foods. You develop a lifestyle that you can live with. You develop a lifestyle that does not leave you with a feeling that you have deprived yourself of anything, and it becomes a habit. Diets just don't work. Diets are something that you go on, and then you go off of. Diets usually force you to deprive yourself of the foods you love. The problem is that when you go off of them, you revert back to the only eating habits you know. You revert back to the bad eating habits that got you overweight in the first place.

A key to losing weight is a lifestyle of balance that becomes a habit. That balance will allow you to have the things you want so you don't feel deprived, balanced with healthier foods for a new way of eating. Then monitor your weight daily to make sure you stay on track. If you want to be thin, don't diet.

Attitude #6: Thin people have positive attitudes.

The sixth attitude of thin people is that they have positive attitudes. You need to have a positive attitude towards yourself. You need to love being thin and be willing to do whatever it takes to stay there. I heard a woman say, "Thin feels better than food tastes." That is a thin person's positive attitude. You need to look at exercise as positive because you love the results. You look at watching what you eat as positive because once again you love the benefits you see from it.

Most overweight people have a bad attitude towards the weight-loss process and towards losing weight itself. It is all about what they have to give up. It is all about the pain and agony of working out. To them, it is not about the benefits they are going to get from exercising. I say it is all about what you focus on. If you want to be thinner you need to focus on the results, not the process. If you want to stay overweight then focus on the pain of the process, not on the positives of the results. Even if you get thin, unless you have a positive attitude towards your new lifestyle, you will never stay thin. This is because having a bad attitude will give you pain daily, and it will pain you every time you have to make the right choice over the easy one.

Attitude #7: Thin people are consistent.

The seventh attitude of a thin person is that they are consistent with both their choices and with their habits.   The other day I had a business meeting with a group of people at an Italian restaurant. It was the type of restaurant that piled up the food. I asked for a carryout container and put some of the food in it immediately.   One thin woman ordered something that was just huge. It was enough for probably two meals, and I jokingly said to her, "I want to see you eat all that," to get a response. She then responded to me very eloquently by saying, "I am not a member of the Clean Plate Club." I responded that I thought her attitude was a great one to have. You need to not be a member of the Clean Plate Club.   She was consistent. That was a choice she made years ago and was consistent about it, and that is one of the reasons she has been thin ever since I have known her. Because she developed the right attitude, she developed the mindset, the thinking that she did not have to clean her plate.

How many of us grew up hearing that we have to clean our plates? What you need to do is **not** be a member of the Clean Plate Club, and that is one of the things that you need to be constant with. You also need to be consistent with exercising.

Last week I had a very intense and busy week. I woke up on Thursday at 5:00 am so I could get my workout in, and for the first time in a while, I just couldn't get out of bed. I dragged myself out of bed anyway, made some coffee, and ate my light breakfast. I was sitting on the chair having my coffee, and I asked myself, "Do I really want to work out this morning?" Just then I caught myself trying to justify not working out, and I laughed and worked out anyway. In the heat of the moment, that thinking can get you in trouble.   Had I planned that week to have one less workout, it would have been fine because it was done in advance. However, to make that decision at the spur of the moment, to make that instant-gratification decision is wrong. It is wrong because it can develop into a bad habit. If I had planned it ahead of time it would have been a conscious decision, not an emotional one. What would happen the next day if I woke up exhausted? Would I skip my workout again? What about the day after that? Would I skip it again? That is why you cannot make instant-gratification decisions. If you are going to cut out a workout, that is fine, but make it a planned decision, not a spur-of-the-moment decision, because that will get you away from being consistent with your workout. Even after years of being thin and working out in the morning, I still am tempted to get off track periodically. Don't let it happen. You need to remain vigilant, you need to remain consistent, and you need to eliminate any bad excuses that creep into your head, or you will find yourself getting off track.

Thin people are consistent. They are consistent with the choices they make daily, they are consistent with their good eating habits, and they are consistent with their exercise.

If you can change your thinking so that you can develop the seven attitudes of a thin person into habits, you too can become and stay thinner.

Summary

Investing in two of your most valuable resources, time and energy, are essential for obtaining anything worth having in life. As a human you have the ability to make daily choices that affect your life, and with these decisions come a great responsibility. I hope and pray that I got you to do one thing: Think!!! I hope I got you to think about what is important to you and how losing weight, getting fit, and adopting a healthy lifestyle can enhance what is truly important to you. I also hope that I have inspired you to take action. I know that you can do it. Make the decision now.

At times in the book I have been direct. This is not because I want to be mean, but because at times all of us need a dose of reality. You are reading this book because you want to lose weight, you want a healthier life, you want a healthier future, and for that I commend you. Follow this with a strong commitment, lots of determination, intense focus, a huge amount of action, and let's get it done. I wish you the best on your weight-loss journey and would like to read about all of your successes.

For more information on weight loss, tools, or to tell me about your successes, please visit http://www.DontDietJustThink.com

Additional Thoughts

Maintain Your New Weight

Weight loss can be categorized into two different mindsets. The first is the mindset needed to lose the initial weight. The second is the mindset needed to maintain the new weight. Both mindsets require a similar yet different way of thinking.

Do you ever wonder why people go through the effort of losing weight just to gain it back within a year? Why is that? The answer is that their thinking has not changed. Once they go off their diets, they return to their old bad eating habits. That is why diets rarely work for the long term. They never changed their thinking. They only changed their bad habits for a short period of time. How will this affect you?

After losing weight, there is an inner battle that continues to go on, trying to pull you back to your previous weight. Watch out and pay attention not to revert back to your old bad thinking and bad habits. Don't let your guard down and don't become complacent or your weight will return. Think of it as a rubber ball. You press down on the rubber ball, and it gets thin. This is because you applied focus and energy to it. This is like what happens when you lose weight. When you take both your focus and your energy off of it, guess what happens to the ball? The ball goes back to its original form. This is the same thing that can happen after you lose weight. After losing the weight you are not done. You are just getting started on your new healthy lifestyle. It still takes focus and energy to maintain and keep you at that new weight. You will still need to monitor your weight daily and take corrective action immediately when your weight goes up. You must challenge any thought that goes against your weight and fitness goals. If you don't challenge your thoughts you will be on the road to failure. It reminds me of the old cartoons that have the devil on one shoulder and the angel on the other, both whispering in your ear. Challenge the guy with the red suit and pitchfork and stay on track. Challenge not only your excuses and justifications but your thinking itself. If there is one thing that I have learned, it is when it comes to your weight, your brain will mislead you whenever it can. It will say things like:

- "Eat it; you can work it off tomorrow."
- "One more won't make much of a difference."
- "I deserve it."
- "I am too tired to work out."
- "It looks so good, eat it!"
- "I'm still hungry, so I'm going up for seconds and thirds."

If your thinking is right, you can win this battle. If you just changed a few habits without the underlying thinking, you will lose this battle.

I want to make it clear, I am not saying never have the foods you like, but remember that you spent a lot of time and energy to lose the weight. Don't lose your focus. Don't lose your determination and don't become complacent. The best thing to do is set another goal (e.g. 6-pack abs, a more toned body, training for a marathon, etc.). Whatever it is, if you set another goal you will tend to stay more focused.

After losing the weight, maintaining it can be easy. You don't need to necessarily continue to make it your primary focus like you did when you lost the weight, but you do need to keep it a close second. It must be on your mind daily. Don't lose weight and forget about it. Always stay focused on your **_Reason Why_**.

Continue to monitor your weight daily and make sure you set a **_Stop Weight_**. This weight is your upper limit. If you hit it, you go into weight loss mode for a day or two so that you can fall back below the **_Stop Weight._** I also recommend staying within a five-pound range. Remembering to step on the scale every day will make it easier to maintain your weight and keep it under control.

Always remember that your weight tomorrow will be determined by the good or bad choices you make today.

Your Health

The ramifications of abusing your body may not be felt for years. If you are overweight or obese and are still in good health, now is the time to act. If you wait until there is a problem before you do something about it, you may be too late. No matter what you think, your body needs to last the rest of your life. It can be a healthy life or a sickly one. I am not saying that just because you are in shape and have a healthy weight you are guaranteed good health. What I am saying is that you optimize your chances of having fewer health problems if you are in shape and have a healthy weight.

If you are overweight or obese, you increase your risk for diabetes, heart disease, stroke, arthritis, and some cancers. Experts say that if you are obese, by losing even five to ten percent of your weight, you can delay or prevent some of these diseases.

On October 31, 2008 the Centers for Disease Control's website had an article with the information below:

"Diabetes is a major cause of morbidity and mortality in the United States, resulting in substantial human and economic costs. National survey data indicate that the incidence of diagnosed diabetes in the United States has increased rapidly and that obesity is a major predictor of diabetes incidence."

"In addition, among 33 participating states with data for both periods, the age-adjusted incidence of diabetes increased 90% from 4.8 per 1,000 in 1995-1997 to 9.1 in 2005-2007."

"Among persons at risk, diabetes can be prevented or delayed by moderate weight loss and increased physical activity. Development and delivery of interventions that result in weight loss and increased physical activity among those at risk are needed to halt the increasing incidence of diabetes in U.S. states."

According to this article, the diabetes rate has almost doubled, but it also said that it can be prevented with weight loss and exercise. Let's think about that.

Although it may taste good, is eating super-sized fast-food lunches, eating bags of chips, drinking beer, or taking seconds at dinner worth getting diabetes, heart disease, stroke, arthritis, or cancer? You have to decide.

I also recently read that the Surgeon General has determined that 70% of all illnesses are due to lifestyle-related causes. These medical costs are attributed to illnesses that could be prevented.

The part about "could be prevented" is interesting. What this is saying is that if people got their thinking right, a lot of these common diseases would become not so common. The great thing is that each of us has the power to control our weight and our fitness. Each of us has the power to make these diseases a thing of the past. Each of us has the responsibility to ourselves and our families to live longer and healthier, to set a good example, and to do our part to reduce the doubling rate of these diseases. Ignoring these statistics and thinking that it will not happen to you is a disaster waiting to happen. Let's think about this and then let's do something positive about it.

Get Fit for Success

Everyone has a different definition of success. Some people view success as power, some as wealth, some as being financially free, some as having great relationships with their family, some as being healthy and fit, some as having a great relationship with their creator. Whatever your definition of success is, health and fitness are a foundation, and it starts with your weight.

If you are religious and you don't take care of yourself and something happens to your health, will it bring you closer to your creator or push you away? Will you become bitter and angry at your creator or will it bring you closer? The relationship will probably change.

Let's look at your family. If you are not in good health, will you have the energy to do the things your family enjoys, or will you be too tired? Will your attitude erode with your energy level? Will you be a grouch that no one wants to be around? It is very difficult to keep a great attitude when you don't feel well, and people don't want to be around people with bad attitudes. If your health fails, will your spouse and children have the pressure and responsibility of taking care of you? How will that affect your marriage and family over time?

Let's look at financial success. There is a computer term, "garbage in, garbage out." This term can also be applied to weight loss and fitness. Whether you are aware of it or not, your body does react to what you put into it. A great example of this is coffee. Millions of people drink coffee in the morning. Why? Because their body reacts to it, and it gives a jump start in the morning. Although on the surface it my not be as noticeable, your body does react to everything you put into it. If you put good food into it your body will react favorably, and will give you more energy and better health. If you eat too much junk, your body will also respond, making you tired all the time and giving you poor health.

Let's look at the example of your car. Would you knowingly buy bad gas for your car? Probably not, but how much bad food do we knowingly put in our bodies that are not good for them? Would you drive your car and never change the oil? What happens to a car you abuse? The sad thing is that some people treat their car better than their body. How does this relate to success, you may ask? If you are not eating right, you probably are not exercising and are most likely overweight or obese. Let's look at how this can affect your success.

After eating a big lunch, how do you feel? Do you want to get up and go or do you want to take a nap? You probably want to take a nap. If you want to eat for success, eat a light lunch: eat fruits and vegetables and get energized instead of sleepy.

I found personally that when I was overweight I had a lower energy level. I also found that I could not maneuver as well as I can now that I am thinner. I need less sleep at night, I can get in and out of the car easier, walk across parking lots faster, and can get more accomplished.

Let's talk about physical appearance. All companies want their employees to make a good impression with their customers. Given that, who do you think they would rather have as a representative of their company, an obese person or a fit person? I am not here to debate the ethical part of this or to say that this is fair. What I will say is that life is not always fair, and you have to deal with it. With that said, perception by your employers and customers could be the difference-maker in your success. I am now thinner, which gives me a neater appearance, which makes a big difference in my businesses.

If you are overweight or obese, statistics say you will have health issues; it is just a matter of time. When this happens it will cost you and your company both time and money. It is hard to become successful if you spend a lot of time in doctors' offices. Companies are also aware of these statistics and whether it is right or wrong they use this information when deciding between two otherwise viable candidates for employment or promotion.

Physical appearance can also affect self-esteem, which is lowered by being overweight or obese. Lower your weight and self-esteem will probably increase. Your appearance also affects your attitude. If you look better, you naturally feel better, and it shows throughout the day. A positive attitude is one of the keys to success. If you don't feel well because of health issues, how do you think it affects your attitude and your energy level? It is difficult to maintain a positive attitude if you don't feel good. It is not easy to go beyond what is expected of you if you don't have the energy. It is hard to keep your focus on your work if you are in pain and worried about your health.

I am not saying that an overweight or obese person can't be successful. There are many examples to prove that incorrect. What I am saying is that they face more challenges than a thinner, fitter person on the road to success. Furthermore, in the long term, thinner and fitter people have better chances of being able to enjoy their success in the long run. Remember two things:

> 1) You cannot enjoy your success if you are not around.
>
> 2) What good is it to have success but lose your health along the way?

Small Bites to Remember

- Place your **Reason Why** on the refrigerator and write it on the bathroom mirrors as your reminder (use a dry-erase marker).
- Don't eat when you have the initial hunger pains. Wait about 45 minutes to an hour, so that the hunger will subside, and you will eat less.
- "Never, never, never, never give up." ~ *Winston Churchill*
- *"Victory belongs to the most persevering." ~ Napoleon*
- Challenge your excuses and challenge your core thinking.
- Identify and eliminate your excuses. Make time for important things.
- A little piece of trivia: The average plate size people used 25 years ago was nine inches. Today most plates are approximately 11 inches. Think about the amount of extra food that we place on those plates.
- Remember that doing nothing about your weight and fitness only hurts you, and your family's future.
- True reality knows where you are and where you want to be.
- Weigh yourself daily and it will keep you focused.
- Tell positive people your goal and the date you will reach it.
- Put a plan together for obstacles or challenges along the way.
- Identify and eliminate bad habits.

Your future weight will be determined by the good or bad choices you make today.

About the Author

As a graduate of Wayne State University with my B.S. in Electrical Engineering, I was trained in solving problems. My first job after college, I developed engineering and manufacturing software for a large automotive manufacturer. In my next position I worked in the same capacity as well as in business systems development for a big automotive supplier. Along the way, I started a computer company that designs systems, fix IT problems, teaches computer skills, and develops software and websites.

Now, what does that have to do with losing weight, you may ask?

Two important things:
1) I applied the same objective problem-solving skills I learned in college to solve my weight problem, lose 50 pounds, and keep it off.
2) I used my experience of analyzing and developing systems to develop a system that anyone who desires to lose weight can use.

Now, add to that the passion I have to teach, and my weight-loss system was born.

Visit

www.DontDietJustThink.com

For

More Weight-Loss Resources

Register Your Book

At

www.DontDietJustThink.com/book

To

Get Your Free Weight-Loss Audio

www.ingramcontent.com/pod-product-compliance
Lightning Source LLC
Chambersburg PA
CBHW072234290326
41934CB00008BA/1297